DIABETES AND ITS MANAGEMENT

Diabetes and its Management

PETER J. WATKINS
MD, FRCP

PAUL L. DRURY
MA, MRCP

KEITH W. TAYLOR
PhD, MRCP

Diabetic Department
King's College Hospital
London

FOURTH EDITION

BLACKWELL SCIENTIFIC PUBLICATIONS

OXFORD LONDON EDINBURGH

BOSTON MELBOURNE

First published 1973
Spanish edition 1974, 1980
Second edition 1975
Third edition 1978
Japanese edition 1983
Fourth edition 1990

Set by Best-set Typesetter, Hong Kong
Printed and bound in Great Britain by
The Alden Press, Oxford

DISTRIBUTORS

Marston Book Services Ltd
PO Box 87
Oxford OX2 0DT
(*Orders*: Tel: 0865 791155
        Fax: 0865 791927
        Telex: 837515)

USA
Year Book Medical Publishers
200 North LaSalle Street
Chicago, Illinois 60601
(*Orders*: Tel: (312) 726–9733)

Canada
The C. V. Mosby Company
5240 Finch Avenue East
Scarborough, Ontario
(*Orders*: Tel: (416) 298–1588)

Australia
Blackwell Scientific Publications
(Australia) Pty Ltd
107 Barry Street
Carlton, Victoria 3053
(*Orders*: Tel: (03) 347–0300)

British Library
Cataloguing in Publication Data

Watkins, Peter J.
    Diabetes and its management. — 4th ed.
    1. Man. Diabetes
    I. Title II. Drury, Paul L. III. Taylor,
    K.W. (Keith William) *1929*
    616.4'62

    ISBN 0-632-02692-8

Contents

Preface to the Fourth Edition

The fourth edition of this book comes over a decade after its predecessor. During that time there have been major advances in knowledge of the aetiology of diabetes. Patient care has undergone radical improvements, diabetes centres are being developed with staff dedicated to the care of patients, and there are many novel techniques in management. Methods for self-monitoring, new methods of treatment to improve control, and glycated haemoglobin assays for assessment of long-term control have been introduced. Treatment of diabetic complications has been given a tremendous new impetus, especially with improvements in foot care and management of renal disease; and dialysis and transplantations are now available to most patients who need them. The availability of laser treatment for retinopathy has increased and the outlook for diabetic pregnancy has improved still further.

So many changes required a new book. Even though it has been completely re-written, our aims remain those of the original authors — namely that it should be of practical help to all those caring for diabetic patients both in hospital and in general practice, and also to the growing number of nurses who have committed themselves to this work. It should also help interested students who would like to expand their knowledge of diabetes beyond that of standard textbooks, as well as registrars and others taking higher examinations. We hope that many others caring for special diabetic problems — obstetricians, ophthalmologists, orthopaedic surgeons and renal physicians — will find helpful information in this book.

Throughout, our inspiration has come from those who first conceived and delivered this book and we hope that the thoughtfulness and wisdom of Dr W. G. Oakley and Dr D. A. Pyke remain permanently in its pages.

Diabetic Department   P. J. Watkins
King's College Hospital   P. L. Drury
London SE5 9RS   K. W. Taylor

Preface to the First Edition

This book has been written as a practical guide to the management of diabetes for the benefit, we hope, of clinicians. It is based on our larger book, *Clinical Diabetes and its Biochemical Basis*, but whereas that was a detailed review of the present state of knowledge concerning all aspects of diabetes, this book is an expression of our own clinical practice. We hope it will be helpful to those with charge of diabetics and also that it will be valuable, either in general practice or in hospital. We hope also that it will be valuable for students who want to know rather more about diabetes than is usually found in general medical textbooks.

Since diabetes affects so many systems, it is the concern of various specialists, for example obstetricians, ophthalmologists, and orthopaedic surgeons, and we trust that they too will find the information they need in this book.

If it is also useful to those taking higher examinations, so much the better.

Diabetic Department   W. G. Oakley
King's College Hospital   D. A. Pyke
London SE5 9RS   K. W. Taylor

Acknowledgments

We are grateful to our colleagues at King's College Hospital with whom we have collaborated over many years, especially Mr Geoffrey Davies, Mr Michael Brudenell, Mr Maelor Thomas, Dr Victor Parsons and Dr David Taube. The Diabetic Clinic staff, together with generations of research fellows and patients, have as ever been a constant source of inspiration. Dr David Leslie kindly contributed the chapter on the diabetic child, Dr Michael Edmonds, whose work on the diabetic foot is well known, contributed greatly to the relevant chapter, Dr Marjorie Doddridge has given invaluable help with the chapter on diabetic pregnancy, and Mr Richard Wilson and his staff helped with that on diet. We are most grateful to Mr Tony Eden for his meticulous proofreading. Miss Gwen Gardner has again typed a major part of the manuscript as she did for the first edition and Mrs Sue Daenen has given tireless energy to bringing the work to completion. Finally, our debt to Mrs Peggy Hinton, our departmental secretary, is enormous.

Section 1
Basic Principles of Diabetes
and its Biochemistry

1: Clinical Presentation, Diagnosis and Classification

Definition

Diabetes is a disorder in which the level of blood glucose is persistently raised above the normal range. It occurs either because of a lack of insulin or because of the presence of factors which oppose the action of insulin. Hyperglycaemia results from insufficient insulin action. There are many associated metabolic abnormalities, notably the development of hyperketonaemia when there is a severe lack of insulin, together with alterations of fatty acids, lipids and protein turnover. Diabetes is a permanent condition in all but a few special situations in which it can be transient.

Background

Diabetes was known in antiquity and remains today a world-wide health problem with a high cost from coronary artery disease, blindness, renal failure and amputations. The scientific basis of diabetes has evolved over centuries; it was long thought to be due to kidney disease, a theory not altered by the discovery of the sweetness of the urine (Thomas Willis, 1621–79) or of glycosuria itself (Matthew Dobson, 1776). The concepts of glucose production by the liver (Claude Bernard, 1813–78) and the discovery that pancreactectomy causes diabetes (von Mering and Minkowsky, Strasbourg, 1889) led to the true scientific understanding of diabetes. After several abortive attempts, Paulesco in Romania (1921) extracted insulin, but it was in Canada also in 1921 that Frederick Banting and Charles Best, together with J. J. R. Macleod and the biochemist James Collip successfully extracted and organized the manufacture and distribution of insulin, sharing the Nobel prize for this great discovery. A 14-year-old boy, Leonard Thompson, was the first patient to be treated in 1922. The major impetus to diabetes treatment and care stems from that date.

The impact of insulin treatment is shown in Fig. 1.1 and is best recorded from Dr Banting's patient, Elizabeth Hughes, aged 14 years. He wrote on 16 August 1922: 'weight 45 lbs, height 5 ft, patient extremely emaciated, slight oedema of ankles, skin dry and scaly, hair brittle and thin, abdomen prominent, shoulders dropped, muscles extremely wasted, subcutaneous

3

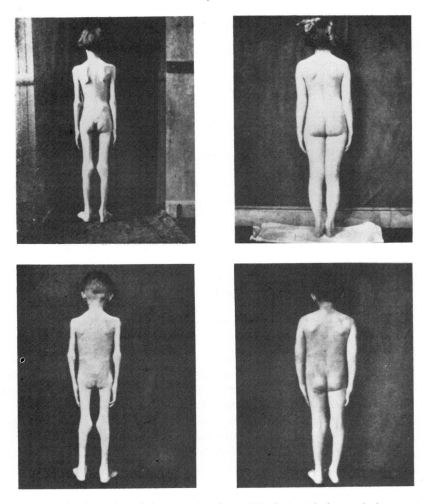

Fig. 1.1 Insulin-dependent diabetes: a view from 1922. Patients before and after starting insulin. (Geyelis, H.R. & Harrop, G. (1922). *Journal of Metabolic Research*, **2**, 767–791).

tissues almost completely absorbed. She was scarcely able to walk on account of weakness'. She started insulin, and 5 weeks later wrote to her mother: 'I look entirely different everybody says, gaining every hour it seems to me in strength and weight . . . it is truly miraculous. Dr Banting considers my progress simply miraculous . . . he brings all these eminent doctors in from all over the world who come to Toronto to see for themselves the workings of this wonderful discovery, and I wish you could see the expression on their faces as they read my charts, they are so astounded in my unheard of progress.'

Classification

Clinical types of diabetes mellitus

The division of diabetes into two major types (Table 1.1) has long been known and over a century ago Bouchardat described patients as having 'diabète gras' or 'diabète maigre'. Bornstein and Lawrence (1951) were the first to show that types of diabetes could be distinguished by the presence or absence of plasma insulin. The distinction between insulin-dependent diabetes (IDD) and non-insulin-dependent diabetes (NIDD) is of immense importance. In practice, many patients need insulin for their well-being but not for survival and this very large group of presumably non-insulin-dependent diabetics blurs the value of this simple and useful classification.

Diabetes has many causes, though most patients have 'primary diabetes' whose aetiology is discussed in Chapter 6. There is a wide variety of conditions which cause secondary diabetes and these are listed in Table 1.1 using the present WHO classification. Individual syndromes are described later in this chapter.

Table 1.1 WHO classification of diabetes

A Clinical classes
  Insulin-dependent diabetes mellitus (IDD)

  Non-insulin-dependent diabetes mellitus (NIDD)
    Non-obese
    Obese

  Malnutrition-related diabetes mellitus (MRDM)

  Other types of diabetes associated with certain conditions and syndromes
    Pancreatic disease
    Disease of hormonal aetiology
    Drug-induced or chemical-induced conditions
    Abnormalities of insulin or its receptors
    Certain genetic syndromes
    Miscellaneous

  Impaired glucose tolerance (IGT)
    Non-obese
    Obese
    Associated with certain conditions and syndromes

  Gestational diabetes mellitus (GDM)

B Statistical risk classes (subjects with normal glucose tolerance but substantially increased risk of developing diabetes)
  Previous abnormality of glucose tolerance

  Potential abnormality of glucose tolerance

Chapter 1

The greatest importance of the present classification (Table 1.1) is the clinical division into IDD and NIDD. IDD is defined in terms of clinical observations and simple investigations (see below) but not by pathogenetic markers; this is not quite synonymous with Type 1 diabetes which is distinguished also by certain genetic and immunological markers, not yet well defined. NIDD (Type 2 diabetes) is present in patients who do not have IDD. Insulin dependence implies a need for insulin injections in order to survive. It is often easy to establish clinically and may be confirmed by demonstrating severe depletion of circulating C-peptide. There are however many middle-aged non-obese patients who need insulin to control symptoms of hyperglycaemia but may not be dependent on it for survival; the exact category is then often difficult to determine.

Malnutrition-related diabetes is now included as a separate category. In tropical countries, young diabetics often present with nutritional deficiency together with diabetes mellitus. The diabetes is often insulin-resistant but without a tendency to ketosis. There may be two important subclasses, namely fibrocalculous (calcific) pancreatic diabetes (see p. 21) and protein-deficient pancreatic diabetes.

Impaired glucose tolerance (IGT) is defined on p. 7. Advice to these patients is discretionary and discussed in Chapter 10. IGT may precede clinical diabetes mellitus. Such individuals have an increased risk of macrovascular disease but are not at risk of microvascular disease.

Gestational diabetes is diagnosed when glucose intolerance is first detected in pregnancy. Reclassification by glucose tolerance test is necessary post-partum. When IGT is discovered in pregnancy it is recommended that patients should be managed in the same way as established diabetics. The diagnostic criteria in pregnancy are the same as those for all adults, though some groups have made alternative recommendations (see p. 194).

The chief importance of the risk category described as 'previous abnormality of glucose tolerance' is the strong likelihood that diabetes will recur under renewed stress, especially from severe infection or other intercurrent illness. This phenomenon is most frequently observed when gestational diabetes returns in subsequent pregnancies.

Diagnosis

Hyperglycaemia must be established in order to make a diagnosis of diabetes. The blood glucose level should be measured using suitable equipment; it is not adequate to use blood glucose strips read by eye. The presence of symptoms with a single random blood glucose value greater than 11.1 mmol/l (capillary whole blood) are together diagnostic of diabetes; if there are no symptoms, there should be at least two elevated blood glucose readings. Diabetes is also likely if a true fasting blood glucose (capillary whole blood) is greater than 6.7 mmol/l. Glycosuria is usually present and provides corroboration for the diagnosis but is itself insufficient evidence.

Diabetes is unlikely if the random blood glucose reading is less than 4.4 mmol/l (capillary whole blood).

When there is doubt about the diagnosis, an oral glucose tolerance test should be performed using a 75 g glucose load (or in children 1.75 g/kg to a maximum of 75 g). It should be performed in the morning after at least 3 days of unrestricted diet and usual physical activity. It is preceded by a 10–16-hour period of fasting during which only water may be drunk. Smoking is not permitted. Intercurrent illness or medication may affect the results and the test should preferably not be performed under such adverse circumstances. Elevated fasting and 2-hour blood glucose levels (Table 1.2) establish the presence of diabetes, without the need for intermediate levels, though these will corroborate the diagnosis. The criteria for IGT are also shown in Table 1.2.

Measurement of blood glucose (or at least a urine glucose test) should be a routine part of medical consultation, especially when the cause of presenting symptoms has not been established, otherwise cases of diabetes will be missed.

'Severity' of diabetes

The terms 'mild' and 'severe' are meaningless and should never be used. Ultimately the only yardstick of 'severity' should be the development of unpleasant complications which occur not just in long-term badly controlled IDD patients but also in some who have never needed any treatment other than diet.

Table 1.2 Glucose tolerance test: WHO diagnostic criteria

	Glucose concentration (mmol/l)		
	Venous whole blood	Capillary whole blood	Venous plasma
Diabetes mellitus			
Fasting	≥6.7	≥6.7	≥7.8
2 h after glucose load	≥10.0	≥11.1	≥11.1
Impaired glucose tolerance			
Fasting	<6.7	<6.7	<7.7
2 h after glucose load	6.7–9.9	7.8–11.0	7.8–11.0

Clinical features identifying IDD

Identifying IDD depends on clinical features as follows: rapid development of classical symptoms of thirst, polyuria and weight loss (over days, weeks or sometimes months) is usual in true IDD patients. They lead to wasting (Fig. 1.1) and physical weakness, and ultimately to vomiting and dehydration. Insulin is always needed urgently. If it is not given, ketoacidosis is inevitable: one-fifth of cases of ketoacidosis develop in previously undiagnosed diabetes whose doctors have usually overlooked their symptoms during preceding weeks. Drowsiness, dehydration and overbreathing (together with acetone in the breath) are the chief features of ketoacidosis which always needs urgent admission and insulin administration.

Clinical presentation

The classical symptoms of diabetes are well known — thirst, polyuria and weight loss combined with pruritus vulvae or balanitis. Patients commonly feel tired and describe striking loss of energy; some develop myopia.

The intensity of these symptoms varies greatly: they tend to be more severe and more acute in IDD than in NIDD patients. The duration of symptoms amongst IDD patients is usually recorded as a few weeks, but it may be as little as a few days or found to extend over several months or longer if a very careful history is taken. At times, transient yet characteristic symptoms are noted with hindsight to have occurred 1 or 2 years previously. Sometimes symptoms appear to begin during intercurrent illness. Transient glycosuria is known to occur occasionally during such illnesses in the pre-diabetic phase, especially in small children. A few patients present in ketoacidosis: this occurs either when the diabetes is very acute in its onset, or much more commonly after two or three visits to a doctor who has failed to recognize the diagnosis of diabetes. These patients usually come to casualty departments weak, thin and dehydrated and with all the features described on p. 97).

The presentation of NIDD patients is in general less acute. They sometimes complain of only one or other of the characteristic symptoms and even then only on careful questioning. Malaise is common and always difficult to diagnose. Symptoms develop over very variable periods, most frequently over several weeks or months, but sometimes they have been treated for long periods, even years, for complaints such as pruritus vulvae without discovery of the true diagnosis. A few patients present with aketotic hyperosmolar coma (but never ketoacidosis, which must be due to IDD) especially when the diagnosis has been overlooked or when patients with intense thirst drink huge volumes of fizzy, sugary fluids.

An increasing number of NIDD patients is found to have diabetes at routine screening examinations when either urine or blood tests are performed. Although some of these patients admit that with hindsight they were aware of characteristic symptoms, many deny them altogether, becoming aware of their previous malaise and loss of energy only after they have received treatment.

Some older NIDD patients present for the first time as a result of diabetic complications; their presence indicates the existence of long-standing unrecognized diabetes which is sometimes confirmed by examination of old medical records and discovery of unnoticed glycosuria or hyperglycaemia years before. Foot sepsis or ulceration presenting in a casualty department almost always indicates a diagnosis of diabetes. Failing vision from cataracts, or less commonly from retinopathy, sometimes leads to the discovery of diabetes. Painful neuropathy rather rarely occurs as a presenting symptom though sensory neuropathy is commoner. Although proteinuria (nephropathy) is not uncommonly present at diagnosis in older patients, diabetes does not normally present with renal failure.

The symptoms of diabetes are so well known that it is surprising that the diagnosis is so often overlooked. It needs to be reiterated that measurement of blood glucose (or a urine test) should now be a routine part of any medical consultation, especially when symptoms have not been accounted for.

Symptoms

Thirst is the most prominent symptom of diabetes and always present in acute IDD. Patients may drink huge volumes of fluid and the use of fizzy drinks with a high sugar content, especially by Afro-Caribbean patients, may cause extreme hyperglycaemia, polyuria and dehydration. Some patients observe that they have a 'dry mouth' but deny thirst and occasionally, when dehydration develops, they may describe difficulty with speech or swallowing. Even this obvious symptom is sometimes overlooked and investigations for speech defects or dysphagia are undertaken.

More commonly dry mouth is ascribed to various drugs (anti-depressants or diuretics in particular) without any thought of the possibility of diabetes. It is interesting that a few patients never seem to develop thirst even in the presence of severe hyperglycaemia.

Polyuria, especially nocturia, is a major symptom and not to be confused with the frequency and urgency of micturition associated with urinary tract infections. Nevertheless many patients are given antibiotics without taking a urine test, and the diagnosis of diabetes is overlooked. The volumes of urine are sometimes huge and cause thirst and eventually dehydration. In the young enuresis, and in the elderly urinary incontinence, may develop as a result of polyuria. Undiagnosed diabetics are often extensively investigated for urological or gynaecological causes of frequency and nocturia before the true diagnosis is made.

Most patients, IDD and NIDD, describe weight loss at the onset of diabetes, which often causes concern at the possibility of some grave disorder. In acute IDD the weight loss is sometimes both acute and profound causing a cadaveric appearance. We have seen many patients whose weight loss has been overlooked and even diagnosed as anorexia nervosa. Weight loss occasionally develops despite a substantial increase in appetite and food intake, especially in the young. Some obsessional patients who keep daily records of their weight throughout life notice weight loss as a very early symptom occurring long before the development of other symptoms of NIDD. Diabetes should always be considered as a potential diagnosis in any patient describing weight loss when no other cause has been discovered.

Fatigue and tiredness are extremely common symptoms of untreated diabetes. They are often attributed by patients to ageing or over-work and frequently accompanied by excessive somnolence and a tendency to fall asleep while watching television. Alleviation of these symptoms by treatment is exceptionally rewarding, many patients describing a new sense of energy and well-being, even those who had previously denied any symptoms at all. Tiredness is not a feature of properly treated diabetes although many patients, usually those with a mild depressive tendency, continue over many years to believe so.

Pruritus vulvae is a presenting symptom of about two-fifths of NIDD women; this, and balanitis in men, is due to monilial infection which occurs in the presence of glycosuria. Doctors often fail to recognize this symptom and patients are frequently treated for symptomatic relief without any thought of the possibility of diabetes. The rash sometimes involves the entire perineum and upper parts of the thighs and may be extremely disagreeable. Balanitis is much less common; it causes some men to go to clinics for sexually transmitted disease before diabetes is diagnosed. Phimosis needing circumcision develops occasionally. Treatment of diabetes and reduction of glycaemia always leads to complete resolution of both pruritus vulvae and balanitis.

The development of myopia at the onset of diabetes is not uncommon; occasionally it is the presenting symptom and astute opticians will send such patients straight to a diabetic clinic (p. 139). Early development of cataract may also cause myopia. Otherwise, deterioration of vision may result from cataract or retinopathy and is the presenting feature in some NIDD patients. Patients should be warned not to return to the optician until the diabetes is controlled.

Physical examination of the diabetic

A full general examination is performed in all cases, whether they are new diabetics or those with long-standing diabetes presenting to a physician for the first time. Newly-presenting IDD patients are often wasted from loss of fat and muscle bulk; they are dry, the tongue is furred and there is sometimes the scent of acetone on the breath. In contrast, there is often a striking absence of physical abnormalities in NIDD patients on initial examination.

Height and weight are documented, and ideal body weight determined. A urine test is always required to establish the presence of glycosuria and whether or not there is proteinuria.

Insulin injection sites should always be examined to discover evidence of fat hypertrophy or more rarely atrophy, or other problems resulting from faulty technique (see Fig. 9.3).

If pruritus vulvae or balanitis are mentioned by the patient, the genitalia should be examined to discover the extent of the monilial rash — it may be very extensive. Balanitis causes an inflamed, cracked and sometimes swollen foreskin which is very unpleasant.

Blood pressure must always be recorded, using a large cuff for the obese.

The fundi are always examined at diagnosis and this must be done through dilated pupils in a darkened room; although retinopathy is rarely present at diagnosis in the young, it becomes increasingly common amongst older patients (see p. 117).

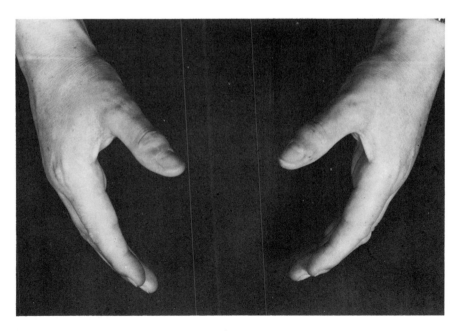

Fig. 1.2 'Cheiroarthropathy': a mild fixed flexion deformity of the fingers is common in patients with long-standing diabetes.

Examination of the feet is important, first to discover any deformities which may need active measures to prevent ulceration; or indeed to discover unreported blisters, ulcers, sepsis or ischaemic lesions of which the patient is unaware. Knee and ankle reflexes are tested to discover the presence of neuropathy, and more detailed sensory examination performed if it is thought to be present. A simple test of vibration perception (see p. 235) is worthwhile and gives a measure of the severity of the neuropathy.

The presence of peripheral vascular disease should be assessed by examination of foot pulses; if both dorsalis pedis and posterior tibial pulses are absent, popliteal and femoral pulses together with evidence of femoral bruits should be sought.

The hands are usually normal, but in those with long-standing diabetes, 'cheiroarthropathy' is quite often seen (Fig. 1.2); this results in a mild fixed curvature of the fingers which makes it impossible to place the hand and fingers flat on a smooth surface. This defect is accompanied by some tightening of the skin over the fingers and is thought to be due to a collagen defect. It causes no disability. Other changes in the hands are due either to median nerve compression (carpal tunnel), or very rarely indeed from severe peripheral neuropathy leading to burns on the fingers similar to those seen in syringomyelia.

THE LIVER

Liver enlargement occasionally occurs in uncontrolled diabetes as a result of fatty (rarely glycogen) infiltration; minor liver dysfunction is sometimes demonstrable. Hepatomegaly resolves completely as diabetes is controlled. Hepatomegaly associated with a slate-grey skin pigmentation is due to haemochromatosis (Chapter 3). It also occurs in patients with the rare conditions of lipoatrophic diabetes and eruptive xanthomata. Hepatic cirrhosis is not itself associated with clinical diabetes mellitus, although insulin resistance, hyperinsulinaemia and glucose intolerance may occur.

SKIN MANIFESTATIONS

Necrobiosis lipoidica diabeticorum (Fig. 1.3) is an uncommon and unsightly blemish of the skin which affects a few diabetic women. It is unrelated to other diabetic complications, or to duration of diabetes, and may even develop before its onset. The shin is the commonest site of involvement, with obviously dilated capillaries (telangiectasis) and a slightly raised pinkish rim; ulceration sometimes occurs. The lesions are indolent, very slowly increase in size and rarely resolve. There is no effective treatment and most women apply cosmetic preparations to ameliorate the appearance of the blemish.

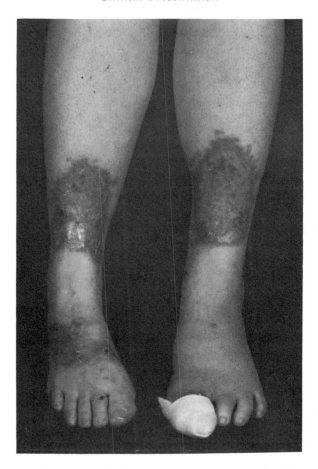

Fig. 1.3 Severe necrobiosis lipoidica affecting the anterior aspects of the legs and right foot.

Granuloma annulare is related histologically to necrobiosis; it consists of a raised pinkish lesion, sometimes in a circular configuration, occurring especially on the hands. Its relationship to diabetes is rather doubtful.

Vitiligo, a common autoimmune disorder causing patchy skin depigmentation, may have an association with IDD.

Eruptive xanthomata are occasionally seen in uncontrolled diabetes, both NIDD and IDD. Crops of multiple 2–5 mm yellowish papules with surrounding pink haloes develop rapidly especially on the elbows, knees and on the buttocks. These changes are associated with exceptionally severe hyperlipidaemia involving all lipid fractions; the serum has a milky appearance, and the retina has an unusual hue sometimes described as 'peaches and cream' associated with very pale arteries and known as lipaemia retinalis. The severe hyperlipidaemia causes spurious lowering of serum sodium which is entirely artefactual. The lesions disappear over a few weeks once the diabetes has been controlled.

Xanthelasmata affecting the eyelids are not a particular feature of diabetes.

Carotenaemia occurs if large quantities of carrots (or pumpkin, sweet potato or tomatoes) are eaten and leads to deposition of carotene in the stratum corneum causing yellow discoloration of soles and palms. Its only association with diabetes is due to the alteration of dietary habit and the excessive consumption of the relevant vegetables.

Other rare skin conditions associated with diabetes are acanthosis nigricans and lipoatrophy, both described in Chapter 3.

Generalized pruritus is not a feature of diabetes and it is very doubtful whether skin sepsis is related to diabetes.

Further reading

Levine R. (1989). Historical development of the theory of pancreatic diabetes. (A translation of the original published in 1929 by O. Minkowski.) *Diabetes*, **38**, 1–6

2: The Epidemiology of Diabetes

The prevalence of diabetes mellitus varies widely between different populations, with a 30-fold variation in incidence between highest and lowest risk countries for IDD and about a 20-fold variation for NIDD. Many population-based studies have shown that, even in Western countries, as many as half of all diabetics remain undiagnosed, though these unidentified cases are all NIDD.

The major factors known to be involved in the varying prevalence of diabetes are age, obesity, genetic background, racial group and geographic region. The relative importance of these differs between IDD and NIDD which will be discussed separately.

The overall prevalence of diabetes in the UK is approximately 1–1.5%, although perhaps 40% of these are unaware of the diagnosis. There have been few good epidemiological studies of IDD in the UK and the information on NIDD relies largely on studies from Bedford and Birmingham in the late 1960s.

Insulin-dependent diabetes

The prevalence of IDD varies some 30-fold between Scandinavia where it is highest and Japan where it is lowest. While the genetic susceptibility to diabetes plays a large part in these differences, there are other significant factors, notably geographical ones. The prevalence of diabetes increases from the equator to the North or South Poles, and there are even trends within Scandinavia (Denmark to Finland), North America (southern USA to Canada) and also in the southern hemisphere within New Zealand (North Island to South Island) (Fig. 2.1). This is consistent with an effect of ambient temperature, presumably via an environmental cause.

The incidence of IDD has been increasing quite rapidly over the past 20 years which provides further evidence for an environmental component. Thus in Finland, the incidence of IDD rose from 13 per 100 000 in the 1950s to 33 per 100 000 in the 1980s. Similar changes have also been noted in Scotland, Poland and North America. Since the incidence of diabetes is increased when children from Japan (a low-risk area) move to Hawaii (a high-risk area), environmental factors of relatively short duration must be present.

15

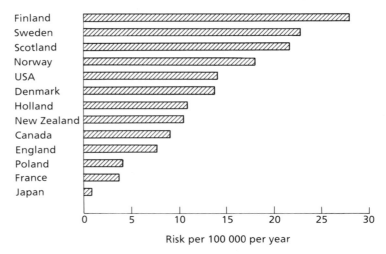

Fig. 2.1 The prevalence of insulin-dependent diabetes in different countries.

The patterns of presentation of IDD are also interesting. The peak incidence is in the early teens for both boys and girls with an increasing incidence from the age of 1 year upwards, decreasing rapidly after the age of 13 years. There is a small male excess. There is also a marked seasonal variation, most cases being diagnosed in the autumn and winter. This again suggests the possibility of a role for environmental causes although, apart from viruses, few serious candidates have emerged.

Genetic risks

As explained in Chapter 6, it is the susceptibility to IDD that is transmitted genetically, not the disease. This is best illustrated by identical twin studies of IDD where only about 30–40% of twin pairs will both develop the disease and become 'concordant'; this contrasts with almost 100% concordance for NIDD. Approximately 1–2% of children of an IDD mother will become insulin-dependent themselves by age 25, the risk appearing to be rather higher if the parent is a father. This represents an approximately 30-fold risk above the general population, but IDD is still an uncommon disease, with total prevalence in the UK of about one in 800 children up to age 16. The risk is higher in the rare instances where both parents have IDD; such couples should be advised to seek genetic counselling although few physicians would discourage pregnancy after full counselling.

As there is no safe or effective method of preventing diabetes in those at high risk, screening procedures are of no value. Indeed, since the majority of new cases are sporadic rather than among siblings or children of known cases, any screening method would have to be applied to the whole population which is obviously impracticable.

Non-insulin-dependent diabetes

Glucose tolerance deteriorates with increasing age among Western populations. The effect is seen in all subjects and does not merely reflect the increasing numbers of diabetics. The effect of age on incidence is dramatic (Fig. 2.2), and perhaps 10% of all European adults above 75 years of age may be diabetic. The lowest recorded prevalences, apart from the Papua New Guinea Highlands where diabetes does not occur, are about 1–1.5% in Third World countries and Eskimos, and the highest about 30–35% in the Pima Indians of Arizona and the islanders of Nauru in the South Pacific.

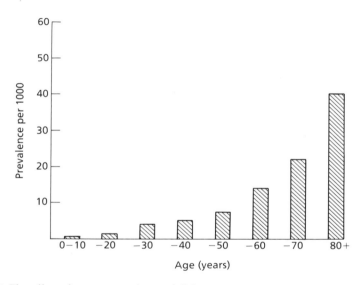

Fig. 2.2 The effect of age on prevalence of diabetes.

The familial tendency to NIDD is poorly understood, though it is obviously very strong with the concordance rate for identical twins (i.e. where both are diabetic) being almost 100%. There is clearly a large genetic role independent of obesity but the mechanism remains obscure.

The prevalence of NIDD increased 2–3-fold between 1960 and 1980 in the USA; there is no comparable information for the UK. Even larger increases have been seen in previously unaccultured groups now taking on a 'Western' way of life.

Role of obesity

Obesity has a major role in the genesis of diabetes. In non-diabetic subjects, glucose tolerance deteriorates as weight increases, with higher fasting and 2-hour post-prandial glucose levels; they sometimes also have higher insulin levels which are insufficient to restore blood glucose to normal. The abnormalities are reversed by weight loss.

Epidemiologically there is a close relationship between the prevalence of obesity and that of diabetes in a population and, in most Western populations, 60% or more of newly presenting patients with NIDD are obese (above 120% of ideal body weight).

Calculations suggest that a subject 25% overweight has a three-fold risk of developing diabetes compared with a normal-weight individual, while one 50% overweight has a 12-fold increased risk.

Racial variations

There are major racial differences in the prevalence of diabetes. The highest known prevalances are amongst the Pima Indians and in Nauru, where gross obesity is also very common. Very high rates of diabetes have also been found in many other specific racial groups; of particular interest and relevance are the following:

1 The Asian population in Southall (Great Britain) has an overall prevalence of diabetes, almost entirely NIDD, of about 2.2%, about four times (when corrected for their younger age) that of the local Caucasian population. This is particularly marked at the ages of 40–65 when the excess above Caucasian rates is as much as five-fold. Recent information suggests that the prevalence is as high among Indians in Delhi.

2 Afro-Caribbean patients in the UK probably also have a slightly higher prevalence of NIDD, again much associated with obesity. The same may be true for American Blacks.

3 Low rates are seen in South African whites and Bantus, while Asian immigrants to South Africa have high rates.

4 The Maltese, Nauruan and Maori populations have high prevalences of NIDD. While part of this may be due to lifestyle, there appear to be underlying genetic risks for diabetes in these groups.

Whatever the underlying mechanisms for these dramatic variations in the prevalence of IDD and NIDD, diabetes is a major public health problem in large areas of the world; a conservative WHO estimate is that there are 30 million diabetics world-wide.

Further reading

Diabetes Epidemiology Research International (1987). Preventing insulin dependent diabetes: the environmental challenge. *British Medical Journal,* **295**, 479–481

Mann J.I., Pyloralala K. & Teuscher A. (1983). *Diabetes in Epidemiological Perspective.* Churchill Livingstone, Edinburgh

Nabarro, J.D.N. (1988). Diabetes in the United Kingdom: some facts and figures. *Diabetic Medicine,* **5**, 816–822

World Health Organization (1985). *Diabetes Mellitus.* Report of a WHO study group. Technical Report No. 727. World Health Organization, Geneva

Zimmet P. (1982). Type 2 (non-insulin-dependent) diabetes: an epidemiological overview. *Diabetologia,* **22**, 399–411

3: Secondary Diabetes, Special Syndromes and Related Endocrine Disease

The many disorders which cause or are associated with secondary diabetes account for a very small proportion of all cases. Diabetes may result from an excess of insulin-antagonistic hormones produced either by disease or administered therapeutically, or from the use of drugs. Several pancreatic disorders are also associated with diabetes and it is a feature of some rare hereditary syndromes. The causes are listed in Table 3.1.

Endocrine causes of diabetes

Corticosteroids and ACTH, growth hormone, glucagon and catecholamines all induce insulin resistance. Patients with tumours producing such hormones often have diabetes.

Cushing's syndrome

Cushing's syndrome of either pituitary, adrenal or ectopic origin is commonly associated with mild diabetes and as many as half of these patients have either overt diabetes or glucose intolerance. It tends to be more common and severe in patients with the ectopic ACTH syndrome, often requiring insulin. Improvement, or cure, of the diabetes occurs when the causative tumour is removed or when satisfactory medical treatment is given, e.g. metyrapone for Cushing's syndrome.

Acromegaly

F. G. Young in the 1930s was able to produce permanent diabetes by giving extracts of growth hormone to dogs. Diabetes, usually mild, is common in patients with acromegaly and occurs in almost one-third of patients, sometimes with quite severe insulin resistance. The diabetes improves after the acromegaly is treated.

Other adrenal causes

Phaeochromocytoma produces similar effects via the catecholamine excess, though classically the glucose intolerance is intermittent. Though primary

Table 3.1 Causes of secondary diabetes

Hormonal	Acromegaly
	Cushing's syndrome
	Phaeochromocytoma
	Glucagonoma
Drug-induced	Corticosteriods
	Diazoxide
Pancreatic disease	Total pancreatectomy
	Pancreatitis
	Fibrocalculous (calcific) pancreatitis
	Carcinoma of the pancreas
	Haemochromatosis
Insulin receptor abnormalities	Lipodystrophy
	Acanthosis nigricans
Genetic syndromes	DIDMOAD syndrome
	Mason syndrome (dominantly inherited NIDD)
Genetic abnormalities of insulin	See p. 55

aldosteronism might be expected to produce glucose intolerance because of the hypokalaemia, this is extremely rare in practice.

Pancreatic diabetes

Diabetes may result from surgical removal or destructive disease of the pancreas (Table 3.1).

Pancreatectomy

Severe IDD always occurs immediately following total pancreatectomy. Because of the concomitant absence of glucagon in these cases, only small doses of insulin are needed and control may be very sensitive to minor changes of dose.

Pancreatitis

Acute pancreatitis can cause diabetes but frequently does not do so; it is usually transient since the amount of pancreatic destruction required to cause permanent diabetes would probably be fatal. Pancreatitis in established diabetes temporarily increases the insulin requirement.

Patients with chronic pancreatitis and cystic fibrosis may develop diabetes. Fibrocalculous pancreatic diabetes, or fibrocalcific pancreatic

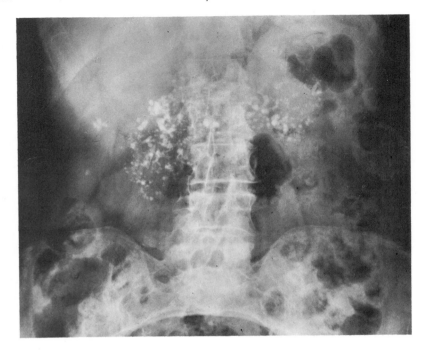

Fig. 3.1 Extensive calcification of the pancreas.

diabetes (Fig. 3.1), occurs in many other areas of the world including India, parts of Africa, Brazil and Indonesia. The disease is identified by the presence of pancreatic calcification seen on a plain abdominal radiography or an ultrasound examination. Some patients with this disease develop steatorrhoea and malabsorption which needs proper investigation and treatment; it is sometimes overlooked and labelled diabetic autonomic diarrhoea from which it must be distinguished. Only five patients attending the King's Diabetic Clinic are known to have this form of pancreatic diabetes, which is rare in Europe and North America.

Carcinoma of the pancreas

There is an association between this disease and diabetes. The cause of the diabetes is obscure since the carcinoma is usually in the head of the pancreas while the majority of islets are in the tail. When patients present with both diabetes and jaundice appearing within a few weeks, pancreatic carcinoma is almost always the cause. Alternatively patients continuing to lose weight after starting treatment for diabetes may prove to have the condition.

Haemochromatosis

This uncommon disease is characterized by a slate-grey skin pigmentation, hepatomegaly, absence of body hair, testicular atrophy, gynaecomastia, impotence, cardiac disease and is sometimes accompanied by arthritis from chondrocalcinosis. It is due to accumulation of iron in the tissues resulting from excessive iron absorption, together with other defects of iron metabolism. The concentration of iron in the liver and pancreas is 50–100 times normal levels. Other endocrine glands also show heavy deposition of iron. Patients are predominantly male (M:F = 9:1) and usually present between 40 and 60 years of age; about two-thirds have diabetes, mostly requiring insulin. Glomerulosclerosis may occur in those patients with very long-standing diabetes. The hypogonadism results from iron overload though occasionally they have hypopituitarism.

The diagnosis is made by demonstrating iron overload (raised serum ferritin and serum iron, saturated serum transferrin) and by liver biopsy which generally distinguishes this condition from the iron overload occurring in some alcoholics. Treatment is by weekly venesection perhaps for 2–3 years, followed by maintenance therapy removing about 2–6 units annually. Hepatic and cardiac failure occur much less commonly after treatment though many patients later succumb to hepatoma.

Transfusion-induced iron overload in some chronic refractory anaemias, for example sickle-cell disease, may also occasionally cause diabetes.

Drug-induced diabetes

Corticosteroids impair glucose tolerance chiefly by increasing gluconeogenesis and increasing insulin resistance. They almost always cause deterioration of diabetic control, often within a few hours of administration. They may precipitate diabetes although they do not normally cause diabetes unless massive doses are used, such as in transplant rejection episodes. Most cases do not remit when steroids are withdrawn. Diabetes is most likely to occur in those who have had a previous abnormality of glucose tolerance or gestational diabetes. Most patients who develop diabetes in relation to steroid treatment can be managed with oral hypoglycaemic agents: established diabetics often require an increase of their treatment and those on large doses of oral therapy quite often require insulin.

Thiazides reduce glucose tolerance by impairing insulin secretion. Diazoxide has the most potent effect and (except in IDD) may cause severe hyperglycaemia, an effect which is sometimes used to advantage in the treatment of insulinoma (p. 215). Thiazide diuretics have a small but still significant hyperglycaemic effect in NIDD and should be avoided wherever possible in diabetics; the action is probably related to potassium depletion.

The combined oestrogen-progestogen oral contraceptive pill has a small effect impairing glucose tolerance. It does not cause diabetes although its use in those who have had gestational diabetes should be carefully monitored. Its effect on diabetic control in established IDD is negligible.

Thyroxine may cause a small deterioration in glucose tolerance: its use does not normally alter diabetic control.

Islet tumours

Glucagonoma

This very rare tumour of the islet glucagon-secreting A-cells is accompanied by characteristic clinical features: these include diabetes, a skin rash (necrolytic migratory erythema), normochromic anaemia and thromboembolic disease. Excision of the tumour leads to a remission of these symptoms. The prognosis when there are hepatic metastases is poor, but improved by chemotherapy.

Somatostatinoma

Most reported cases of this exceptionally rare D-cell tumour of the islets have been associated with diabetes. Insulin, glucagon, pancreatic polypeptide and growth hormone levels are all reduced. Diagnosis is usually made late in the course of the disease.

Insulinoma

See chapter 20.

Other causes and hereditary causes of diabetes

Lipoatrophic diabetes

'Lipodystrophy and hepatomegaly with diabetes, lipaemia and other metabolic disturbances' was first described by Lawrence who later named the syndrome lipoatrophic diabetes. It is a very rare condition which affects both sexes and, in half the cases described, developed before the age of 16. It is characterized by generalized, complete lipodystrophy, lipaemia with cutaneous xanthomata, hepatomegaly and insulin-resistant diabetes. It carries a bad prognosis and death is due to hepatic failure, gastric haemorrhage or intercurrent infection.

There is an association between acanthosis nigricans (pigmentation affecting axillae and groin, associated with a velvety skin), lipoatrophy and extreme insulin-resistant diabetes resulting from an absence of insulin receptors.

DIDMOAD syndrome (diabetes insipidus, diabetes mellitus, optic atrophy, deafness)

This is a recessively inherited syndrome in which IDD is associated with the development of diabetes insipidus, optic atrophy leading to blindness, and gradual onset of high-tone deafness. Many of these patients also have distended bladders with hydroureter and hydronephrosis.

Mason syndrome (dominantly inherited NIDD)

This syndrome was named after the propositus. NIDD occurs in at least three generations, the pattern indicating a dominant pattern of inheritance. The diabetes has its onset in youth and it is striking that it remains non-insulin-requiring over many decades. Long-term diabetic complications may occur less frequently, and in some families there is also evidence of a low renal threshold for glucose. There is no HLA association. The family tree of the original Mason family is shown in Fig. 3.2.

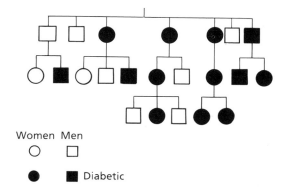

Women Men
○ □
● ■ Diabetic

Fig. 3.2 The family tree of the Mason family showing dominant inheritance of NIDD.

Other hereditary syndromes

There are nearly 50 genetic syndromes associated with impairment of glucose tolerance or clinical diabetes. These include pancreatic degenerative syndromes, haematological conditions, metabolic abnormalities, neurological syndromes and often chromosomal abnormalities. The better known syndromes include:

1 Friedreich's ataxia.
2 Klinefelter's syndrome.
3 Turner's syndrome.
4 Dystrophia myotonica.
5 Refsum's syndrome.
6 Laurence–Moon–Biedl syndrome.
7 Werner's syndrome is a rare condition characterized by premature ageing, hypogonadism and scleroderma, together with diabetes in about half the cases.

Other endocrine diseases and diabetes

Other autoimmune disorders including thyroid disease, pernicious anaemia and Addison's disease are also associated with IDD. Less often ovarian, testicular and pituitary antibodies may be present (Table 3.2).

Table 3.2 Organ-specific autoimmune diseases associated with IDD

Antibody to	Disease association
Islet cell	IDD
Thyroid microsomes ⎱ Thyroglobulin ⎰	Primary hypothyroidism
Gastric parietal cell	Atrophic gastritis
Intrinsic factor	Pernicious anaemia
Adrenal cortex	Addison's disease
Ovary	Premature ovarian failure
Testis	Primary testicular failure

Hypopituitarism and diabetes

Bernardo Houssay described in the 1930s the amelioration of diabetes following hypophysectomy. Control of diabetes after hypophysectomy may be difficult requiring very small doses of insulin and patients may be sensitive to small changes of insulin dose; they are at great risk of severe hypoglycaemia. A decrease of insulin requirement also occurs with the spontaneous development of hypopituitarism in cases of Sheehan's syndrome which may occur either suddenly or over several years. Indeed a falling insulin requirement may alert the physician to the diagnosis.

Addison's disease

Addison's disease, which is much commoner in IDD then in the general population, usually presents with gradual onset of malaise, skin pigmentation, hypotension and diarrhoea, with diminishing insulin requirements and a tendency to hypoglycaemia.

Thyroid disease

Thyrotoxicosis has a small adverse effect on glucose tolerance and causes a relatively slight upset in established diabetes, although there are exceptions when the tendency to ketosis is greatly increased. Thyrotoxicosis is sometimes detected at a very early stage in those regularly attending a diabetic clinic by the insidious and initially unexplained loss of weight.

The effects of primary hypothyroidism on diabetes are very slight: it is however a very common disorder and frequent cause of ill-health. Thyroxine and TSH should be measured if there is any doubt as the condition may be difficult to detect, especially in younger patients.

Further reading

Dymock I.W., Cassar J., Pyke D.A., Oakley W.G. & Williams R. (1972). Observations on the pathogenesis, complications and treatment of diabetes in 115 cases of haemochromatosis. *American Journal of Medicine*, **52**, 203

Tattersall R.B. (1974). Mild familial diabetes with dominant inheritance. *Quarterly Journal of Medicine*, **43**, 339

4: The Pancreas, Insulin Secretion and Action

Properties of insulin and its structure

Insulin was rapidly produced with considerable purity soon after its discovery, although its structure was not determined until the 1950s, when Frederick Sanger demonstrated its amino acid sequence. This work, for which Sanger was awarded a Nobel prize, was especially important since insulin was the first protein to be sequenced.

It is a small protein (molecular weight 5700), containing only 51 amino acids arranged in two chains and joined by sulphur links (Fig. 4.1). The amino acids are shown in detail because there are small changes in the sequence in different species. Thus pig (porcine) insulin is almost identical with human insulin, differing only in the terminal amino acid of the B-chain which is alanine in the pig instead of threonine in man. Such small changes in structure do not usually have significant effects on the biological activity of insulins but it is these differences which are partially responsible for antibody production. Treatment of diabetes is now increasingly with human insulin.

Insulin is also a very stable protein. It is not easily destroyed by heat, although enzymes in the gastrointestinal tract will quite rapidly break it down making its oral administration impossible.

Since the exact amino acid sequence of many insulins is now known, it is natural to speculate on specific areas of the molecule which could be associated with its biological activity, for example by combining with receptors. Extensive studies on insulin crystals (using X-ray crystallography) have suggested that the last few amino acids of the B-chain (on the left hand side of Fig. 4.1) are especially important. Indeed a substitution of one of these amino acids by mutational change is known to occur in some families in the United States as a rare genetic disorder. This change is accompanied by mild diabetes. In this sense genetic change among the insulins resembles mutations among the haemoglobins though mutational change among insulins is a very rare cause of diabetes.

Structure of the islets of Langerhans and insulin release

In mammals the islets consist principally of B-cells which are responsible for synthesizing and secreting insulin. A much smaller proportion of cells

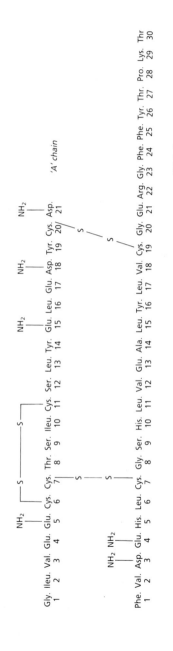

Fig. 4.1 Amino acid sequence of human insulin.

synthesize the other main pancreatic hormone, glucagon. These are known as A2-cells. In addition very small quantities of other hormones may be made in the islets. These include somatostatin, a very short peptide which inhibits the release of a number of hormones, and pancreatic polypeptide. The general structure of an islet is shown in Fig. 4.2. The distribution of islets within the pancreas is not uniform; islets containing predominantly B-cells are concentrated in the tail.

Within the islet both the B-cells and the A2-cells contain large numbers of granules in which both insulin and glucagon are stored (Fig. 4.2). When secretion takes place, these granules move to the plasma membrane of the cell and discharge their contents into the blood. Glucose is the main substance which triggers this release process, although it can also be

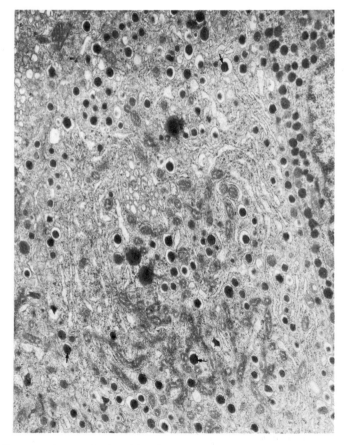

Fig. 4.2 Electron micrograph of an islet showing insulin granules.

modified by drugs such as the sulphonylureas. The biochemical mechanism which enables the B cells to respond in this way is a complicated one and is now the subject of intense experimental investigation. It is, however, known that glucose has to be oxidized within the B-cells for release to take place. Moreover, a rise in B-cell intracellular calcium ion concentration is also necessary, as is an increase in the messenger substance cyclic AMP.

The secretory process is disturbed in some types of disease. It is also grossly deranged in tumours of the islets of Langerhans, where an unregulated secretion of insulin may take place leading to profound hypoglycaemia.

A more direct way to study insulin release is to measure the output from individual islets incubated with glucose. In most mammals a sigmoidal type of curve is obtained; this is also true for human islets as shown in Fig. 4.3.

The shape of this curve means that very little insulin is released at low glucose concentrations (below 5 mmol/l) but, as glucose concentration is increased, the release of insulin is accelerated dramatically with maximal release seen at approximately 15 mmol/l. It is this mechanism which ensures that the blood glucose remains within very narrow limits. Any rise in blood glucose following the ingestion of food will lead to a corresponding extra release of insulin into the circulation as a compensatory mechanism. So important is this homeostatic mechanism that any disturbance in it due to disease will lead to major disturbances in metabolism. Thus a defective release of insulin in response to glucose appears to underlie much of NIDD. These defects are discussed further on p. 44.

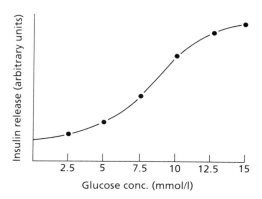

Fig. 4.3 Response of isolated islets to glucose stimulation (from Wallis M., Howell S.L., & Taylor K.W. (1985). *Biochemistry of the Polypeptide Hormones*, p. 270. Wiley-Interscience, Chichester).

Alterations in blood insulin after glucose stimulation

In man, insulin release can be studied by infusing glucose into a peripheral vein. The response to IV glucose is shown in Fig. 4.4. Plasma insulin is measured at various times after the infusion; in normal individuals the islets respond with a sharp rise in blood insulin.

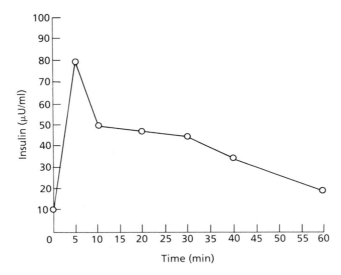

Fig. 4.4 Insulin response to intravenous glucose in normal man (from Wallis M., Howell S.L. & Taylor K.W. (1985). *Biochemistry of the Polypeptide Hormones*, p. 270. Wiley-Interscience, Chichester).

The response to oral glucose (the oral glucose tolerance test, OGTT) is slower and the return to normal insulin levels delayed. The actual height of the response is very much dependent on the amount of oral glucose, now standardized at 75 g for an adult. Fig. 4.5 shows such a response in normal individuals. If the total output of insulin is measured after oral glucose this is seen to be considerably greater than the response to an equal amount of glucose infused intravenously. This augmentation of the effect of glucose by mouth is usually interpreted as a consequence of gastrointestinal hormones liberated in the wall of the gut due to the presence of glucose. Such hormonal factors travel in the portal blood to the islet cells to liberate more insulin.

Other factors stimulating insulin release

Apart from glucose the most important physiological agents promoting release are amino acids — especially arginine and leucine. This means that

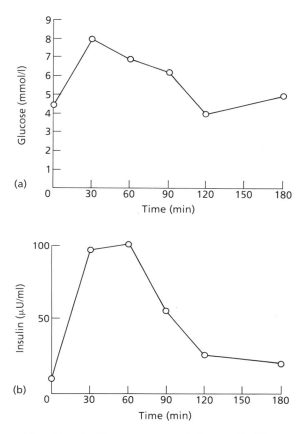

Fig. 4.5 Glucose (a) and insulin (b) response to oral glucose (75 g) in normal man.

following the digestion of a protein meal extra insulin will be secreted. This additional insulin rapidly depresses blood amino acid levels by ensuring their transport into cells, and by increasing protein synthesis. Infusion of amino acids such as arginine or leucine is sometimes used as a test of islet function.

Among drugs increasing insulin release, the most important are those of the sulphonylurea group, which are extensively used in the treatment of NIDD. They may function by altering the balance of calcium ions within B-cells.

B-cell function is also altered in conditions where extensive physiological change takes place, such as in pregnancy and during growth in the child. Both pituitary growth hormone and placental hormones increase the responsiveness of islets to glucose, so that more insulin is produced both during growth and towards the latter part of pregnancy. In some women there is an inability of the B-cell to respond to the need for extra insulin and temporary diabetes (gestational diabetes) ensues.

Factors diminishing insulin release

The hormone adrenaline inhibits insulin release, and this may be important in helping to conserve blood glucose during exercise. Insulin release is also greatly diminished during starvation when the B-cells of the islets become less sensitive to glucose stimulation.

Insulin biosynthesis

Insulin, like other polypeptide hormones, is made as a higher molecular weight precursor. The immediate precursor of insulin called 'proinsulin' is a single chain substance. This is split just before granule formulation into insulin itself and a short peptide termed the connecting peptide (C-peptide). Both the newly formed insulin and C-peptide coexist within the B-cell granules (Fig. 4.6). Both are released into the circulation, molecule for molecule. Indeed the measurement of C-peptide can give a very reliable index of the secretory function of islet B-cells, if measurement of insulin in blood is made difficult. This is the case when insulin antibodies are present, as they usually are after the treatment of patients with beef (bovine) insulins. Moreover, in the case of insulin-producing tumours, relatively large quantities of proinsulin may also be simultaneously released into the circulation.

Production of human insulin by genetic manipulation techniques

Human insulin is now most usually produced by methods which are based on the use of recombinant DNA in bacteria. The basis of the method is the

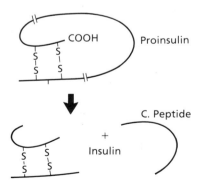

Fig. 4.6 The biosynthesis of insulin.

introduction of the human insulin gene into bacteria. The bacterial protein synthesis system can then be switched on to make human insulins, or more strictly their precursors, in bulk — the extraction of insulin from such preparations is a relatively simple matter. The insulin gene itself, which is necessary to start the process, can either be made from messenger RNA extracted from the pancreas, or can be synthesized chemically.

Glucagon

Glucagon is the other major hormone of metabolic importance present in the islets of Langerhans. It is present in the A2-cells, although substances of rather similar chemical structure are also produced elsewhere in the gastrointestinal tract. Glucagon has a smaller molecular weight than insulin (3400) and is a single chain polypeptide. Like insulin it is present in granules although unlike insulin its release is triggered by low glucose concentrations. Its principal activity in man is to raise blood glucose by increasing hepatic gluconeogenesis, and it is therefore of importance during fasting or hypoglycaemia. It is also sometimes used therapeutically to combat extreme hypoglycaemia; its effect is dependent on adequate hepatic glycogen stores.

Mode of action of insulin

Insulin is the most important polypeptide hormone which regulates metabolism in mammals and its absence results in severe, and ultimately fatal, diabetes. Glucagon is less essential, in man and some higher animals, although it is of major importance in some reptiles and birds.

The action of insulin can be summarized by stating that it is essential for the biosynthesis of large molecules such as glycogen, triglyceride and protein from small molecules such as sugars or amino acids. Thus, although the most clinically obvious effect of insulin is its effect in the lowering of blood glucose, it also produces profound effects on the deposition of fat and

Table 4.1 The major effects of insulin

Insulin *increases*	Glucose transport (muscle)
	Glycogen synthesis (muscle and liver)
	Fat synthesis (adipose tissue)
	Protein synthesis (muscle and other tissues)
Insulin *decreases*	Gluconeogenesis (liver)
	Fat breakdown

the synthesis of body protein. It is necessary in growth and in pregnancy, both of which are marked by the laying down of extra protein. The principal tissues on which insulin is effective are muscle, adipose tissue, and liver. It does not affect brain tissue or red blood cells.

It will be seen that insulin controls a very wide range of biochemical activities, which are summarized in Table 4.1.

Effects on carbohydrate and fat metabolism

In most mammals, the intravenous administration of insulin will result in the lowering of blood glucose within minutes. How is this effect achieved?

The earliest consequence is an increase in glucose transport in tissues such as muscle and adipose tissue. This effect is on the sugar transporting systems in the plasma membrane. What happens to the glucose once inside the cell depends very much on the type of tissue. In muscle, insulin increases activity of the enzyme glycogen synthetase which increases glycogen deposition. Most of the glucose rapidly disappearing after insulin administration can be accounted for in this way. In adipose tissue (which lacks glycogen) insulin increases the deposition of fat.

Fat is stored as triglyceride (Fig. 4.7) which consists chemically of glycerol and fatty acid. Both glycerol and fatty acid are ultimately derived from the breakdown of glucose. Insulin, in fact, increases the activity of a number of enzymes involved in the breakdown of glucose by glycolysis, and in the synthesis of fatty acids. Hence fat deposition is considerably increased. This is why the feeding of excessive amounts of carbohydrate results (after digestion) in a rise in blood glucose which in turn stimulates the islets to secrete more insulin.

Stored fat does not persist within adipose tissue as an inert material, as was once thought. It is constantly undergoing breakdown and re-synthesis from fatty acids and glycerol. The enzymes which break down fats in this way are termed lipases — their mode of action is shown in Fig. 4.7. The

Fig. 4.7 Action of a lipase.

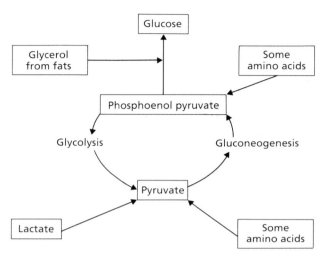

Fig. 4.8 Pathways of gluconeogenesis.

breakdown of stored fat under the influence of a lipase is the first step leading to ketosis. Insulin inhibits the activity of adipose tissue lipase and hence suppresses triglyceride breakdown, and ultimately ketosis.

Effects on protein synthesis

As already indicated insulin increases protein synthesis. This effect is at the level of the ribosomes and is still not well understood. Insulin can be properly considered as a growth hormone whose action is distinct from that of pituitary growth hormone itself, which is thought to act through insulin-like growth factors.

Effects on gluconeogenesis (Fig. 4.8)

Gluconeogenesis is the process by which small molecules such as amino acids and lactate are converted to glucose in the liver. Amino acids are in turn derived from the breakdown of protein, so that gluconeogenesis provides a mechanism for the conversion of protein into carbohydrate, and specifically into glucose. This process is of great importance during fasting when muscle wasting may be obvious.

The actual pathway by which amino acids are converted to glucose is a complicated one. It is not simply a reversal of the normal glucose

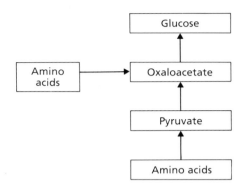

Fig. 4.9 Metabolism of amino acids leading to glucose production (gluconeogenesis).

breakdown pathway (glycolysis). The intraconversions are shown very diagrammatically in Fig. 4.9.

Insulin inhibits the activity of several important enzymes in the gluconeogenesis pathway and therefore turns the process off. The effect of insulin in inhibiting gluconeogenesis further reduces blood glucose; conversely insulin deficiency will lead to increased gluconeogenesis.

Insulin action at the cellular level

Is there any simple explanation for the way in which insulin produces this multiplicity of events? Despite many years of intensive research, no single mechanism provides a satisfactory answer. It is certain, however, that before insulin can affect any aspect of metabolism, it has first to combine with a receptor on the surface of the cell membrane. The first event which follows the attachment of insulin to it is the combination of a phosphate group with the insulin receptor protein. Subsequent events leading to the activation of enzymes are still unclear.

The number of receptors on the cell surface for insulin also seems to vary. This fluctuation in receptor number is an important way in which the action of insulin may be modified.

Mode of action of glucagon

Glucagon raises blood glucose by breaking down liver glycogen. It does so by activating the enzyme phosphorylase and thus increases gluconeogenesis. It is often, therefore, termed a hormone of glucose need and it is released in greater quantities during fasting in man. It is generally believed to act entirely by raising cyclic AMP in cells.

Further reading

Alberts A., Bray D., Lewis J., Raff M., Roberts K. & Watson J.D. (1989). *Molecular Biology of the Cell*. Garland Publishing Company, New York

Draznin B., Melmed S., LeRoith D. (eds.) (1988). *Molecular and Cellular Biology of Diabetes Mellitus. Vol II, Insulin Action*. A.R. Liss Inc., New York

Wallis M., Howell S.L. & Taylor K.W. (1985). *The Biochemistry of the Polypeptide Hormones*. John Wiley, Chichester

5: Control of Blood Glucose and the Biochemistry of Diabetes

The general factors which affect blood glucose are:
1 The rate of absorption of carbohydrate from the gastrointestinal tract.
2 The rate at which glucose is released into the blood from the liver.
3 The rate of glucose utilization in the peripheral tissues.

The rate of absorption from the gut depends upon the nature and frequency of meals. The rate at which the liver releases glucose into the blood depends both on liver glycogen breakdown and on gluconeogenesis. Glucose utilization is affected by several external factors including exercise. Hormones of various kinds modify all these processes. The effects of insulin have been discussed in the preceding chapter.

Effects of non-pancreatic hormones on metabolism

Insulin is the only hormone which lowers blood glucose. By contrast, adrenaline, corticosteroids, growth hormone and glucagon can all increase the levels of circulating glucose. The metabolic balance between insulin and other hormones is therefore of great importance in maintaining blood glucose within narrow limits (usually between 3 and 7 mmol/l). Diseases of other endocrine glands apart from the islets of Langerhans may cause widespread disturbances of metabolism which include diabetes.

Adrenaline

Adrenaline from the adrenal medulla rapidly increases blood glucose concentration by breaking down liver glycogen. It does so by activating the enzyme phosphorylase. This is presumed to be the major mechanism by which intense fear can provoke a temporary hyperglycaemia. Adrenaline also inhibits insulin release.

Adrenal steroids

Cortisol (the major product of the adrenal cortex) raises blood glucose by increasing gluconeogenesis. It is particularly important in the longer-term regulation of metabolism, when it is effective by increasing the levels of key enzymes, which promote gluconeogenesis in liver tissue.

Growth hormone

Pituitary growth hormone administered to some animals produces diabetes. Moreover the association between the disease acromegaly and diabetes has long been documented. Excessive amounts of growth hormone can directly damage the B-cells of the islets by a process which is not properly understood.

Under physiological conditions, growth hormone acts as a major hormone increasing protein synthesis. However, under fasting conditions, it acts as an anti-insulin hormone. This is achieved by increasing fat breakdown. In turn, fatty acids liberated from adipose tissue may slow down glycolysis. Consequently, acromegalics may show insulin resistance. By contrast, in hypopituitarism, there is often extreme sensitivity to the action of insulin, due to the absence of growth hormone.

Effects of meals and of fasting

Following a meal containing carbohydrate (or protein), insulin output from the B-cells of the islets will be increased. This will ensure that there is a rapid transfer of glucose to tissues and the synthesis of liver and muscle glycogen as well as of triglyceride. By contrast, in fasting, the lack of food, either carbohydrate or protein, results in a fall in blood insulin. The earliest consequence is a breakdown of liver glycogen. This takes place after even an overnight fast in man. If fasting continues, both fat and protein stores are catabolized to provide energy. Fatty acids are used as a fuel, and they may also spare the utilization of glucose; gluconeogenesis is also increased. On account of these elaborate control mechanisms, the blood glucose will rarely fall below 3.0 mmol/l even in quite prolonged fasting.

Biochemical changes associated with IDD

It has been known for many years that, in IDD, the islets of Langerhans are reduced in number and show distinct types of histological change. In some individuals, most of the islets may have disappeared, and been replaced by fibrous tissue. A careful study of the insulin content in the pancreas from such patients reveals that insulin may be almost entirely absent. It is clear that in many cases of IDD there is an absolute deficiency of insulin.

A similar situation may be seen in experimental animals following administration of substances highly toxic to the B-cells of the islets, such as alloxan or streptozotocin.

The most evident metabolic changes seen in IDD are hyperglycaemia and ketosis. In addition, wasting of body protein and fat may also be obvious, particularly if the condition has been prolonged. Hyperglycaemia is associated with intense polyuria, and the ketosis with a serious metabolic acidosis. The hyperglycaemia may be very considerable, and values as high as 100 mmol/l have been recorded in untreated cases. More usually the figures at diagnosis range from 15 to 80 mmol/l. The blood ketones are considerably more elevated than they are in starvation. Total ketones may be as high as 30 mmol/l in diabetic ketoacidosis, compared with about 8 mmol/l in prolonged starvation.

These changes are all the results of severe insulin deficiency. They are summarized in Fig. 5.1. Insulin deficiency depresses glucose transport and glycogen synthesis in tissues such as muscle. Due to the defective activity of a number of enzymes in the glycolysis pathway, glucose utilization is slowed. At the same time there is a depression of protein synthesis, and a corresponding increase in protein breakdown. Lack of insulin switches on the enzymes in liver which promote gluconeogenesis. Amino acids derived from protein will therefore be converted to glucose with greater facility. Overproduction of glucose from this source complements glucose underutilization.

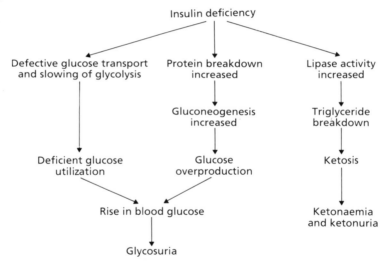

Fig. 5.1 Metabolic consequences of insulin deficiency.

The increased breakdown of fat also directly follows as a consequence of insulin deficiency. A low blood insulin results in increased lipase activity in adipose tissue cells. Long-chain fatty acids so released are transported in the blood to the liver. Within the liver, they are broken down to yield large quantities of acetyl-coenzyme A. Some of this, instead of being burnt by the tricarboxylic acid cycle, is diverted to the formation of acetoacetate (Fig. 5.2). Acetoacetate is easily decarboxylated to give acetone or alternatively is

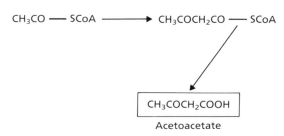

Fig. 5.2 The formation of acetoacetate in liver.

reduced to form β-hydroxybutyrate (Fig. 5.3). Collectively, acetone, aceto-acetate and β-hydroxybutyrate are known as the ketone bodies. Neither acetoacetate nor β-hydroxybutyrate are inert materials. Both are rapidly metabolized by many tissues to provide considerable amounts of energy, although large quantities of these substances are excreted in the urine. Acetone, which is volatile, is excreted both in the breath and in the urine. Until quite recently, acetone was regarded as being non-metabolizable, and was thought of as an inert end product. Very recent work has, however, shown that as much as 20% of acetone produced in human diabetic ketosis is converted to glucose or lactate.

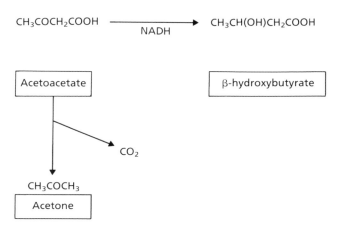

Fig. 5.3 Formation of ketone bodies.

Some secondary consequences of hyperglycaemia and ketosis in IDD

Hyperglycaemia results in a massive loss of glucose in the urine as the renal threshold for glucose is exceeded. This is accompanied by a large loss of body water, and therefore by dehydration. Ions, such as Na^+ and Mg^{2+} are also lost in quantity in the urine. In the absence of insulin, potassium leaks from cells and plasma potassium may rise. In addition to increased blood acetoacetate and β-hydroxybutyrate, blood lactate and long-chain fatty acids are also increased.

Collectively these all contribute to produce a severe metabolic acidosis, in which the blood pH may fall to as low as 6.8. (The fluid and electrolyte changes in diabetic ketosis, and their management, are dealt with in Chapter 11 in greater detail.)

Biochemical changes associated with NIDD

Cases of NIDD usually present with an apparent lack of clinical ketosis though blood ketone levels in this condition are still increased above the normal range.

It has been more difficult to explain in biochemical terms the changes which are associated with NIDD. In this condition some pancreatic insulin is present, though not as much as for normal subjects — there is therefore only a partial loss of islet function. The pattern of insulin release in a non-obese patient with NIDD following oral glucose is shown in Fig. 5.4. Despite the hyperstimulation of the islets by a high blood glucose concentration, the response is less than normal and is delayed, and there is generally a deficit in insulin secretion. If the blood glucose is allowed to rise in this group of

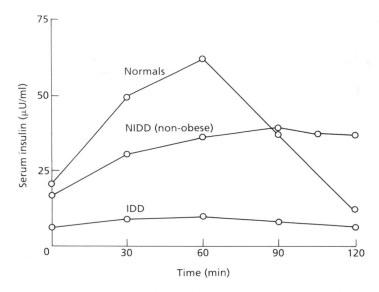

Fig. 5.4 Insulin responses after 50 g glucose. Results for normal subjects and ketotic diabetics are shown for comparison.

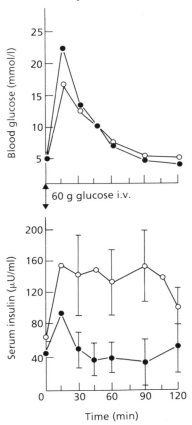

Fig. 5.5 Insulin and glucose response in normal and non-diabetic subjects following intravenous glucose (from Karam J.H. *et al.* (1963). *Diabetes*, **12**, 197). o, Obese group (3 ♂, 7 ♀; ●, normal group (5 ♂, 3 ♀.)

patients, then the insulin response may be considerable though still less than is seen in normal subjects whose blood glucose is artificially raised to comparable levels.

In addition, there is ample evidence of insulin resistance in this group of patients. By insulin resistance is implied an insensitivity to the action of insulin such that a much greater concentration of insulin is needed to exert a particular biological effect. This may affect the liver, muscle and adipose tissue. Insulin resistance is particularly associated with obesity.

A physiological example of resistance is seen in the last trimester of pregnancy, where insulin resistance is usually encountered. Normal women secrete more insulin at this time in order to overcome the resistance, while IDD women need larger doses of insulin than earlier in pregnancy (Chapter 18).

The effects of obesity in increasing insulin resistance are illustrated in Fig. 5.5. Here is shown the plasma insulin response to intravenous glucose in normal people and non-diabetic obese individuals. More insulin is needed to normalize the blood glucose.

The mechanism for the insulin resistance of obesity is still imperfectly understood. One reason for resistance is a reduced number of receptors in tissues due to high circulating insulin levels. High hormone concentrations suppress the number of hormone receptors present on the plasma membrane of cells ('down regulation'). In addition, there is also evidence for a defect in the mechanism for coupling the action of the receptor to subsequent biochemical events (a 'post-receptor' defect).

It has already been suggested that the islets in NIDD are relatively insensitive in their response to glucose. The additional stress on the islet imposed by obesity may well result in diabetes.

Some other effects of chronic hyperglycaemia

The sorbitol pathway

In prolonged hyperglycaemia, the metabolism of glucose is diverted away from glycolysis into the production of sorbitol; the enzyme involved is an aldose reductase. The sorbitol so produced may be further metabolized to yield fructose (Fig. 5.6). Frequently, the rate of production of sorbitol is excessive and a high concentration of this may accumulate in the lens, brain and nerves as it does not readily pass out of cells. In the eye, this may be related to cataract formation. In the nerves, where excessive quantities of

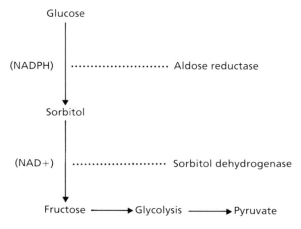

Fig. 5.6 The sorbitol pathway.

glucose may also be present in addition to sorbitol, it has been supposed that the presence of these two sugars is related to diabetic neuropathy.

This accumulation of sorbitol in diabetic tissues gives a rationale for the use of aldose reductase inhibitors in the treatment of diabetic neuropathy (Chapter 15).

Protein glycation

An increased chemical association of glucose with proteins is seen in prolonged hyperglycaemia. Apart from haemoglobin, several other proteins such as fibrin or albumin may be affected. The reaction with haemoglobin which takes place in red cells has been particularly studied. Here glucose reacts with the terminal valine residue of one of the chains of haemoglobin. After a rather complex series of reactions, a ketoamine, haemoglobin $A1_c$ ($HbA1_c$), is produced (Fig. 5.7).

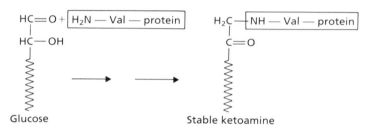

Glucose   Stable ketoamine

Fig. 5.7 Formation of glycated haemoglobin.

The formation of $HbA1_c$ is highly dependent on glucose concentration, and its measurement is now frequently used as an index of overall diabetic control (Chapter 7).

Further reading

Taylor R. & Agius T. (1988). The biochemistry of diabetes. *Biochemical Journal,* **250,** 625–640

6: Aetiology and Pathogenesis of Diabetes

There have been tremendous advances in understanding the mechanisms which may cause diabetes, especially IDD, although the precise causes are still not known. The following describes the most important recent advances.

Pathology of the pancreas

There are striking differences in the changes occurring in IDD and NIDD. The most characteristic changes develop in IDD, in which B-cells disappear, and the insulin content and numbers of islets are drastically reduced; negligible amounts of insulin can be extracted from the pancreas in this type of diabetes (Fig. 6.1). Insulitis is seen in some of these cases but not in NIDD. In contrast, the pancreas in NIDD may contain normal numbers of islets, and extractable insulin may be little different from normal; the finding of amyloid in these islets is of great interest. In this condition subtle biochemical changes must be present which prevent the normal insulin response to a glucose stimulus.

Insulin-dependent diabetes

SELECTIVE B-CELL LOSS

The selective destruction of B-cells may occur due to an autoimmune process, as a result of virus infection or from exposure to toxic chemicals. Some B-cells do however persist, though in small numbers, in about half of people with IDD of less than 10 years duration, and in 10% of those of longer duration. Evidence for B-cell regeneration is very scarce but can be found in those who have died soon after diagnosis.

LYMPHOCYTIC INFILTRATION (INSULITIS)

An infiltration of lymphocytes in or around the islets is the most characteristic change in IDD and one which is in keeping with an immune process (Fig. 6.2). It is found most frequently in children who have died suddenly soon after the onset of diabetes but it is not common, occurring in

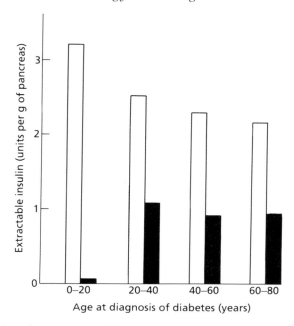

Fig. 6.1 Variation of average extractable insulin at post-mortem extract in diabetics (black) with age at diagnosis. Values for non-diabetic controls shown in white (from Wrenshall G.A., Bogoch A. & Ritchie R.C. (1952). *Diabetes*, **1**, 87).

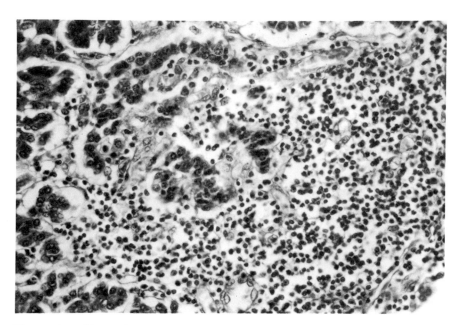

Fig. 6.2 An infiltrate of lymphocytes around an islet in a case of IDD.

under 15% of pancreases examined, and up to 40% of those under 5 years of age. Insulitis affects only a few islets, and is rarely seen after a diabetes duration of more than 6 months.

FIBROSIS

Some islets appear to be replaced by fibrous tissue, although glucagon and somatostatin cells may still be present. These findings are inconstant.

Non-insulin-dependent diabetes

The appearance of the islets in NIDD are not necessarily different from those in non-diabetics. However, the deposition of hyaline material in the islets was first described by Opie in 1901. Endothelial cells appear to be responsible for this amyloid-like substance which, in some instances, may entirely replace a B-cell. It is not pathognomonic for diabetes: it is rare under 40 years of age, but present in about half of the diabetics over 70 years old. Recently the structure of this amyloid material has been described; its precise role is disputed.

Pathogenesis of IDD

If IDD is generally associated with the extensive destruction of the B-cells, what are the likely factors responsible for this change? Most opinion now considers them to be a combination of environmental and genetic factors which are in turn associated with an autoimmune response to the islets.

Evidence of the operation of environmental factors on the aetiology of the IDD comes from many virus studies, from observation of the effects of some toxic chemicals and from the changing geographical incidence of IDD. A distinct seasonal variation in the incidence of IDD has also been observed.

Toxic chemicals

Ever since the discovery of the highly diabetogenic chemical, alloxan, in the 1940s, there has been continuing interest in chemicals which destroy the B-cells. Alloxan was originally described as a substance which was toxic to the renal tubules in animals. Later it became clear that it also destroyed the B-cells of islets. It has been extensively used to produce an insulin deficient diabetes in animals. Despite extensive investigation, there is no evidence to incriminate it as a cause of diabetes in man. Streptozotocin, which is a nitroso-derivative, behaves similarly to alloxan although it is more selective in its effects on the B-cells. Both these substances may give rise to islet cell antibodies. Quite recently, diabetes has been induced in man as a result of contact with the rodenticide 'vacor'. The diabetes induced by this substance is again insulin-dependent, although it is accompanied by a severe peripheral neuropathy. There has also been a suggestion from Iceland that smoked mutton may cause diabetes. Several drugs toxic to the islets and used in the treatment of other conditions may induce diabetes, usually NIDD. Among them are thiazide diuretics and especially diazoxide, used in the treatment of hypertension. The effects of this drug are freely reversible; it has been used in the treatment of insulin-secreting tumours.

Viruses

The suggestion that viruses are in some way implicated in the destructive processes in the islets which lead to diabetes is not new. The possibility that mumps is involved was raised in the middle of the last century. More recently, rubella virus and members of the Coxsackie B group have been postulated as diabetogenic viruses in man. While the evidence for implicating Coxsackie B viruses in a few cases is now good, it is still uncertain whether most patients with IDD have suffered a predisposing virus attack.

MUMPS

Diabetes due to mumps is a rare event in the UK. Furthermore, the widespread use of mumps vaccine has not noticeably diminished the incidence of IDD in those countries in which it has been used. In some northern European countries, however, notably Finland, there has been very recent evidence of a more specific association of preceding mumps infection with diabetes.

RUBELLA

Surveys conducted both in Australia and in the USA showed that the offspring of mothers who had acquired rubella in pregnancy were much more likely to develop diabetes, often as late as the third decade of life. The diabetes was both IDD and NIDD in type, and was sometimes accompanied by the presence of islet cell antibodies. The mechanism by which a virus can induce these long-term effects is clearly of great interest.

CYTOMEGALOVIRUS

There is some evidence for the occasional association of this DNA virus with diabetes, but it seems unlikely to be a common antecedent of IDD.

COXSACKIE AND RELATED PICORNA VIRUSES

The sera of people newly diagnosed with IDD may contain higher titres of antibody to Coxsackie B4 than that of controls. Further evidence for Coxsackie involvement has come from cases of overwhelming Coxsackie infection. In two cases, viruses isolated from the patients induced diabetes in mice. Research in animals has indicated that only certain strains of Coxsackie B4 are diabetogenic and such strains may be relatively uncommon in man, where they arise by virus mutation.

Very recently, minor disturbances of glucose tolerance and islet cell antibodies have been found among children in Cuba following an outbreak of Echo 4 virus infection. Echo 4 virus is closely related to Coxsackie viruses.

VIRUSES WHICH CAUSE DIABETES IN ANIMALS

The case for a viral factor in the aetiology of clinical diabetes is also supported by a large number of experimental models in which diabetes has been produced by viruses in animals. At least 20 viruses are at present known which attack the islets of Langerhans in animals. Prominent among these viruses are the small RNA viruses known as the picorna group. Diabetes definitely attributable to a virus was first noted in cattle during an outbreak of foot-and-mouth disease in southern Italy; foot-and-mouth disease virus is a member of this group. Another picorna virus, EMC virus (encephalomyocarditis virus), may produce severe diabetes in mice. Experimentally such viruses may disrupt insulin synthesis and release.

How may such viruses function so as to cause diabetes? They may cause an immediate destruction of B-cells by a cytolytic process, which is however likely to be a rare event. Alternatively they may induce longer term changes including the initiation of an autoimmune response directed against islets.

Seasonal incidence of IDD

Gamble was the first person in the UK to demonstrate conclusively that IDD showed a marked seasonal incidence with a peak incidence in the autumn and winter months. Since then similar relationships have been shown in several other parts of the world, including the southern hemisphere. The reason for this observation is still unclear. It might represent the unmasking of a latent diabetes by non-specific virus infection. On the other hand, it may represent a more specific virus attack on the islets.

THE CHANGING PATTERN OF IDD IN OTHER COUNTRIES

Further evidence for a role of environmental factors in the aetiology of diabetes is seen in the changing incidence of diabetes with time in some European countries (see p. 15).

Genetic aspects of IDD

That patients tend to have a family history of diabetes has been known for many centuries and has been repeatedly recorded by physicians. The exact mode of inheritance, however, is complex and not completely understood, not least because of the heterogeneity of diabetes itself. It is now clear that it is factors which predispose to IDD which are inherited, rather than IDD itself. Recent studies on the insulin gene and on the immune system, as well as on the twins of diabetics, have done much to clarify the situation.

In the UK approximately 20% of all people with IDD have a positive family history with at least one first-degree relative affected by the disease. The corollary to this is that the majority of diabetics do not have a first-degree relative with diabetes. The chances of the child of an IDD patient developing the disease at some time are increased many times compared with the children of unaffected individuals (Chapter 18). With better methods of genetic analysis, it may be possible to improve prediction in the future. There are a few rare syndromes in which many members of a family may be affected. These and other very rare syndromes are discussed elsewhere (p. 25).

STUDIES ON TWINS

Studies on identical twins provide particularly valuable information on the relative roles of genetics and the environment in the pathogenesis of diabetes. The largest and most remarkable of such studies was conducted by Pyke and his colleagues and now includes over 300 pairs of identical twins, one or both of whom have diabetes. The most important findings in this group relate to concordance rates among the major classes of diabetics. More than half of the IDD twins were discordant (i.e. only one had diabetes), showing that genetic factors cannot be the sole cause of diabetes. By comparison there is almost complete concordance in the NIDD identical twins (i.e. both have diabetes) which implies that genetic factors are the chief determinants of this condition.

The unaffected twin of an IDD patient may however display lymphocyte abnormalities which disappear with time. These abnormalities include an increase in the number of activated T-lymphocytes. Mild but persistent metabolic abnormalities have also been recorded in this unaffected group. These observations are consistent with the possibility that some common environmental factor may have initially affected both twins, although only one twin shows changes progressing to total B-cell destruction.

THE BART'S WINDSOR STUDY

This famous family study was established by the late Professor Andrew Cudworth. HLA genotyping of all families in the Windsor area who had a child with IDD and at least one unaffected sibling was undertaken. Susceptible individuals proved to be those with the haplotypes in common with the proband (affected child). Complement-fixing islet cell antibodies were found only in genetically-susceptible groups, although diabetes has only developed in about half of them so far. Antibodies were present for months or even years before the onset of diabetes, indicating that development of insulitis is a very gradual process; minor and intermittent changes in random blood glucose were also seen well before development of diabetes. Disappearance and reappearance of islet cell antibodies was also observed.

INHERITED ABNORMALITIES OF THE IMMUNE SYSTEM: THE HLA SYSTEM

The major histocompatibility antigens (MHCs) are adjuncts to several types of immunological activity. They are glycoproteins present on the surface of cells, and they are coded by genes on the short arm of chromosome 6. In man, the major histocompatibility antigens are termed HLA antigens (or human leucocyte-associated antigens, since they were originally found on human leucocytes). They are subdivided into three main groups. Thus, class I MHC molecules are needed for the lysis of cells infected with viruses, and they are present on all cells. Class II molecules (e.g. HLA-DR) have a more limited distribution and are necessary for the activity of T-helper cells. Class III molecules are associated with the action of complement. An association of Class I antigens (HLA-B8 and B15) with IDD was first described more than a decade ago; but more recently Class 2 antigens (HLA-DR3 and DR4) have been found to be much more closely associated. More than 90% of IDD patients show either DR3, DR4 or both together; the relative risks are shown in Table 6.1. In contrast DR2 appears to be protective against diabetes.

These haplotypes are of course common in the general population, 60% possessing either DR3 or DR4, and are in no sense specific for diabetes. Attempts have therefore been made to examine the association with several subsets of either DR3 or DR4; the discovery of a very close association with the DQβ gene is important, and furthermore, the recent identification of single amino acid abnormality of this gene in those with IDD is very exciting. There is also some association of IDD with the complement (Class

Table 6.1 Relative risk for IDD associated with HLA-DR genotypes

HLA-DR genotype	Relative risk
DR3 alone	3
DR4 alone	5
DR3 and DR4	14
DR2	0.4

III) genes which play an important part in clearance of immune complexes and viral neutralization. In particular C4 levels are reduced in IDD as a result of non-expressed genes. Other complex associations have been described.

These HLA associations with IDD apply only to northern European populations; other associations are gradually being described in different racial groups.

THE INSULIN GENE

The structure of the insulin gene which is located on the short arm of chromosome 11, is now known in detail. Changes in the structure of the gene itself may lead to the manufacture of abnormal insulins, similarly to the production of abnormal haemoglobins. There are only a very few instances in which insulins with an abnormal structure have been produced, and when diabetes develops it has been very mild and never IDD. More abnormal insulins are likely to be described in the future. Changes in the sequence of nucleotides flanking the gene, on the other hand, have been recorded much more commonly than in control subjects. This is especially so for IDD. These changes could determine the rate at which insulin is produced; while such changes may be important as markers for diabetes, their functional significance is dubious at present.

Autoimmunity and IDD

CIRCULATING ANTIBODIES TO ISLETS

The possibility that an autoimmune response could be associated with the onset of diabetes was suggested by the lymphocytic infiltration sometimes seen at post-mortem around the islets in IDD. In the 1970s antibodies against islets were detected in the serum of diabetic patients who had other autoimmune endocrine disorders. Most patients with IDD are now known to have circulating islet cell antibodies although the titre of these decline during the first 12 months after presentation. Circulating antibodies to islet cells include complement-fixing antibodies, some of which are specific for the B-cell, and islet cell surface antibodies which react with the A-, D- or B-cells in the islets. These antibodies may appear in the sera months or years before the onset of the disease; they are identified particularly in genetically-predisposed relatives of diabetic patients. Not all patients who possess islet cell antibodies develop diabetes; even though patients with complement-fixing antibodies are very likely to develop diabetes, there is still no method of predicting its development in any individual. Complement-fixing antibodies are also found in diabetes associated with other autoimmune endocrine disorders in whom they tend to persist.

What is the role of such antibodies in mediating changes leading to B-cell destruction? There are reports which suggest that such antibodies may impair insulin release or synthesis. Direct cytotoxicity of islets in culture as seen *in vitro* is not necessarily relevant to the situation *in vivo*. However, since islet function is normàl in some patients with islet cell antibodies, they might only represent markers of damage from some other cause.

INSULIN AUTOANTIBODIES

Quite recently the appearance of autoantibodies to the insulin molecule itself has been described in newly diagnosed IDD patients. These antibodies, which are normally present in low titre, have to be distinguished from those insulin antibodies induced by the injection of insulin from different species into patients in the course of treatment. Autoantibodies do not appear to have any physiological significance, but may appear before the onset of clinical diabetes. They too may indicate previous islet cell damage.

CELLULAR IMMUNITY

Apart from possible damage by circulating antibodies, the effects of different classes of inflammatory cells may also be important. These include cytotoxic T-cells, and macrophages (which can produce lymphokines) as well as natural killer cells. The mode of action of these cells is complex and often involves the participation of cell surface glycoproteins, namely the major histocompatibility antigens (MHCs) already described.

Cellular events at the onset of diabetes are difficult to study, except in the rare instance of the death of an IDD patient during development of the disease. Indirect methods of study, for example by examining peripheral lymphocytes, are therefore undertaken and have shown a marked increase in the number of activated lymphocytes in the blood of patients with newly diagnosed IDD.

An alternative approach is to use animal models. The best known of these is the BB (or Biobreeding) rat. This mutant animal develops diabetes after 60–120 days associated with marked insulitis. There is marked hyperglycaemia, and ketosis. Transfer of lymphocytes from afflicted rats to normal rats results in transfer of the diabetes. Clearly, in these animals, cell-mediated destruction of B-cells results in diabetes.

EFFECTS OF IMMUNOSUPPRESSION IN THE PREVENTION OF IDD

Because of the immunological changes associated with the onset of IDD, attempts have been made to prevent it by immunosuppression. While immunosuppression can successfully reverse the diabetes of the BB rat, results have been less encouraging in man so far. Initial attempts with steroids with or without azathioprine were unsuccessful, but there is now clear.evidence that cyclosporin A will produce a remission (avoiding insulin use) in a small proportion of patients started within 6 weeks of diagnosis. Unfortunately the benefit is only present as long as cyclosporin is continued; indeed it may be lost despite continued therapy, and there are unacceptable side effects, notably renal impairment and hirsuties. Clinical use is therefore unjustifiable and attempts are continuing to develop an alternative effective agent with less toxicity.

The value of any such agent however requires the very early diagnosis of diabetes, and requires identification of those about to develop the disease if it is to be widely effective in preventing IDD. However the observation that some islet function can be preserved by immunosuppression is clearly of the greatest importance in understanding the cause of diabetes and has very exciting implications for the future.

Conclusions

Selective loss of B-cells in the islets of the pancreas is the cause of IDD. It is an insidious process triggered by an unknown stimulus which probably leads to an insulitis and the appearances of islet cell antibodies. These events take place months or perhaps years before the development of clinical diabetes. They occur predominantly in genetically-predisposed individuals who usually show the HLA haplotype DR3 or DR4, with an even stronger association with DQ; those with DR2 are relatively protected. It is not yet possible to predict which individual will develop diabetes, but if this becomes practicable, the future of immunosuppression in preventing diabetes may one day become a reality.

Chapter 6

Non-insulin-dependent diabetes

AETIOLOGY OF NIDD

NIDD represents a heterogenous group of disorders and has many different underlying causes, few of which are well understood. Most of these are described in other parts of this book, but are summarized here. Secondary causes are discussed in Chapter 3.

NIDD has a strong genetic basis (see p. 53), usually polygenic and poorly understood; no genetic markers are known. Autosomal dominant inheritance is responsible in a few families ('Mason-type' diabetes, see p. 25). Twin studies have shown that nearly all identical twin pairs are concordant (i.e. both twins are diabetic) in contrast to IDD where many twin pairs are discordant for diabetes (p. 53). A family history for diabetes is also more likely amongst NIDD than IDD twins. NIDD is also associated with several genetic syndromes.

Insulin secretion is disturbed in the majority of NIDD patients (p. 44). First-phase (i.e. immediate) insulin response is usually impaired or absent, and most NIDD patients have reduced insulin levels during insulin tolerance tests, at least as compared with equally hyperglycaemic non-diabetic subjects. Apparent hyperinsulinaemia in some cases may be accounted for by an increased proportion of proinsulin which has been described using newer methods of insulin assay. These important changes in insulin secretion are accompanied by a relatively modest decrease in islet B-cells; the role of amyloid found in the islets of some NIDD patients remains to be determined (p. 51).

Impaired sensitivity is probably an important factor in the development of NIDD although its relative importance compared with that of B-cell dysfunction is unclear. The mechanism of insulin resistance however remains obscure; insulin receptor numbers and affinity may be abnormal but such defects vary considerably in different tissues and their aetiological role remains uncertain.

Mutant insulins (p. 55) may cause hyperinsulinism and, very occasionally, NIDD. Other abnormalities might include those of insulin receptor genes, glucose transporter genes, or genes for diabetes related peptide (amyloid, p. 51), and there may be abnormal restriction length polymorphisms.

Environmental factors may also play a role in causing NIDD. While dietary factors alone do not cause diabetes, obesity is strongly related to NIDD (p. 18) and physical inactivity may be an additional factor. The increasing incidence of NIDD with age and racial variations are described on p. 18.

Further reading

Barnett A.H. (ed) (1987). *The Immunogenetics of Insulin-Dependent Diabetes.* MTP Press, Lancaster

Barnett A.H., Eff C., Leslie R.D.G. & Pyke D.A. (1981). Diabetes in identical twins: a study of 200 pairs. *Diabetologia*, **26**, 87–93

Diabetes Epidemiology Research International (1987). Preventing insulin-dependent diabetes: the environmental challenge. *British Medical Journal*, **295**, 479–481

Leslie R.D.G., Lazarus N.R. & Vergani D. (1989). Events leading to insulin-dependent diabetes. *Clinical Science*, **76**, 119–124

Tarn A.C. *et al.* (1988). Predicting insulin-dependent diabetes. *Lancet*, **i**, 845–850

Section 2
Principles of Treatment

7: An Overview of Management

Objectives

The aims of treatment are primarily to save life and alleviate symptoms. Secondary aims are, as far as possible, to prevent long-term diabetic complications and, by eliminating various risk factors, to increase longevity. The first aim is relatively easy to attain and in some elderly patients or those who lack motivation or ability it is the only aim.

Control of diabetes is achieved either by diet alone, or diet with oral hypoglycaemic agents or insulin. Insulin-dependent patients are often in need of urgent treatment which should be started without delay; identification of patients who need insulin treatment is described in detail on pp. 8 & 74. Most other patients should start their treatment with dietary measures alone, after proper confirmation of the diagnosis by blood glucose measurement; oral hypoglycaemics are not usually given until dietary treatment has failed. Treatment of IDD patients is always more urgent than that of NIDD patients; they must be referred very quickly, sometimes on the same day.

Control of diabetes should reach the best standard which can reasonably be achieved for an individual person. Once symptoms have been eliminated, well-being improved and weight corrected, careful consideration must be given to the need for 'tight' control. The aim of trying to obtain blood glucose levels close to normal is to attempt prevention of long-term complications; the evidence that this might be possible is discussed elsewhere (see p. 116). The price of 'tight' control is often a devastating frequency of disabling hypoglycaemic attacks. Furthermore, some patients become disabled in a different way by making the goal of 'tight control' their main aim and effort in life which is taken over by an obsession with their condition.

Common sense must prevail and patients not always criticized if tests are less than perfect. That said, many patients, especially pregnant women, are able to maintain astonishingly good control of diabetes using modern methods of insulin administration and monitoring.

Risk factors which shorten life should be reduced as far as possible: advice to stop smoking and control of hypertension are the most important of these. Reduction of obesity is desirable, and treatment of hyperlipidaemias should be undertaken when appropriate (Chapter 16).

Proper education is an essential part of management and should include instruction about diabetes and its treatment as well as prevention of some of the complications of diabetes, notably foot problems.

Management must obviously include systems for screening and treatment of diabetic complications. These are discussed in the appropriate chapters.

Assessment of diabetic control

Several factors need to be assessed to determine whether treatment is adequate.

SYMPTOMS

Symptoms should be assessed; if they are still present treatment is inadequate. However, their absence does not necessarily indicate good control of diabetes. Indeed, some patients who have suffered chronic hyperglycaemia may for a time feel worse when the blood glucose is reduced.

WEIGHT CHANGE

This must be assessed at every consultation. If control is poor and weight is decreasing, more intensive treatment is needed. On the other hand, if weight gain is recorded in the presence of poor control, then the patient is almost certainly overeating. There is also the obvious aim of reducing obesity as a general health measure as well as a part of diabetes management; body mass indices (kg/m^2) of more than 27 for men or 26 for women are regarded as unsatisfactory.

BLOOD GLUCOSE MEASUREMENT

Blood glucose measurement by the patient is now the chief yardstick by which to assess treatment; it is particularly important for insulin-treated patients so that they can identify peaks and troughs of blood glucose, enabling them to make appropriate adjustments of treatment. Blood glucose profiles should be recorded in a suitable book which is brought to the clinic consultations. For NIDD patients, the blood glucose levels for which to aim are less than 8–10 mmol/l post-prandially or less than 6 mmol/l fasting. For IDD patients more flexibility is needed because of the greater swings of blood glucose, but most should be in the range of 4–10 mmol/l; this is discussed in more detail on p. 83.

URINE TESTING

This is still useful for those who cannot manage to perform blood glucose measurements. Two tests are performed:

1 *For glucose*: dip-stick tests are very simple and also cheap. Urine testing is therefore still valuable for many patients who cannot perform blood glucose measurements and especially helpful for NIDD patients on whom tests should be glucose-free most of the time. Urine tests for IDD patients have some role to complement blood glucose readings, although they can be variable and not very informative. As blood glucose measurements become simpler and more reliable, one would expect fewer patients to rely on urine testing.

2 *For ketones*: patients do not generally need to test urine for ketones; although some find it helpful when hyperglycaemia develops, most are confused by the results since ketonuria is quite a common finding especially in morning samples from young IDD patients.

GLYCATED HAEMOGLOBIN (HbA1)

Glucose is bound to haemoglobin after its synthesis leading to the formation of glycated haemoglobin, or haemoglobin A1, which is composed chiefly of haemoglobin $A1_c$ together with small amounts of haemoglobin $A1_a$ and $A1_b$. Persistent hyperglycaemia modifies haemoglobin A at a constant rate during the life of the red blood cell so that the level of haemoglobin A reflects the overall blood glucose control during the previous 4–6 weeks. The use of HbA1 measurement to assess diabetic control is now a standard procedure. The normal range (Corning method, see Appendix) is 5–8%; in practice it is quite difficult to achieve this ideal (normal) level of HbA1 of less than 8% and it is adequate to aim for less than 9.5%. Even this may be difficult for some patients especially those with IDD, and higher levels may have to be accepted.

Spurious HbA1 levels are recorded in some conditions especially when abnormal haemoglobins are present or red cell turnover is altered. HbA1 is thus sometimes increased where HbF is present because some methods of measurement cannot distinguish it from HbA1, and in haemolytic anaemias, falsely low readings may be obtained.

Other glycated proteins have been measured and suggested as markers of diabetic control. Fructosamine has the advantage of rapidity and inexpensiveness but is not sufficiently reliable, and glycated albumin represents too short a period of hyperglycaemia to be of particular value.

LIPIDS

Hyperlipidaemia is common in uncontrolled diabetics (see p. 167). It is not worthwhile making lipid measurements until optimal management has been achieved; i.e. diabetes and weight controlled, and smoking preferably stopped. Then assessment of blood lipids will reveal those who have persistant hyperlipidaemia perhaps requiring treatment (see p. 168).

Conclusions

Management of patients with diabetes aims to save life, eliminate symptoms and in the long-term to reduce complications and other risk factors which may shorten life, especially smoking and hypertension. Specific treatment for the diabetes itself needs proper advice and education which are paramount. Assessment of diabetic control is undertaken by appraisal of symptoms and weight changes, review of home blood or urine glucose tests together with clinic blood glucose and HbA1 measurement. Lipids are measured when appropriate control has been achieved. Arrangements need to be made for screening and treatment of diabetic complications.

Further reading

Refer to main textbooks and see general reading list on p. 240.

8: Dietary Principles in Diabetes

Successful dieting is the key to successful diabetic treatment. Indeed, in the era before insulin was available, the very vigorous carbohydrate-free starvation diets had a profound effect not only on symptoms but on the course of the diabetes itself.

The aims of dieting are to reduce blood glucose thereby decreasing symptoms; to ensure optimal weight, focusing therefore on reduction of obesity; and to ensure adequate growth in children. Diet needs to be tailored to suit individual patients and their habits in terms of physique, occupation, cultural habits and religious beliefs. A good dietetic service is essential for diabetes care and in the first instance at least, advice must be given individually; subsequently diet teaching for groups of patients becomes very important. Unrealistic advice will not be followed; this is especially important for those working with ethnic minority groups who must be aware of the relevant dietary habits.

General advice

Elimination of simple, rapidly absorbed sugars (sucrose and glucose) is the minimum requirement for all diabetics. It is difficult to obtain adequate diabetic control unless this is done. Simple sugars are used only for

Table 8.1 Simple dietary instructions

Do not eat or drink:

Sugar or glucose in any form and do not use sugar in your cooking
Jam, marmalade, honey, syrup or lemon curd
Sweets or chocolates
Cakes and sweet biscuits
Tinned fruit
Lucozade, Ribena, Coca-cola, Pepsi-cola, lemonade and other fizzy drinks

Apart from these foods and drinks, you may eat and drink anything else, just as you did
   before you were diabetic

You may use artificial sweeteners, such as saccharin, Sweetex, Hermesetas, Saxin, but
   not Sucron, and any sugar-free drinks including squashes and slimline ranges

---

treatment of hypoglycaemia. In some older patients with NIDD this measure alone will often suffice with minimal disruption of lifestyle; a card showing the simplest dietary instructions is shown in Table 8.1. For obese patients, the energy supply must be restricted in order to reduce weight at least towards the ideal.

The carbohydrate (starch, polysaccharide) content of diabetic diets is more liberal now than in previous generations, and those which are highest in their fibre content have the least hyperglycaemic effects. Carbohydrate still needs to be controlled, however, and most diabetics are aware of the deterioration in control when they overeat. The fat content of diets should be reduced in order to minimize adverse effects on development of coronary artery disease, and polyunsaturated fats rather than saturated fats are probably of benefit. Current policies recommend that more than 50% of the calorie content should be from carbohydrate and that fat should not contribute more than 35%; these rigorous recommendations represent ideals which are not easy to achieve.

The fibre content of food comes either from the foodstuff itself or can be added as guar gum from Indian cluster beans. Storage polysaccharides (galactomannans) of legumes, and pectins of cell walls, especially of fruits, are rich in their fibre content. Wholemeal bread, wholemeal breakfast cereal, nuts, fresh fruit and vegetables are all rich in fibre; such foods are listed in Table 8.2.

Table 8.2 High-fibre foods

Bread	Wholemeal or stoneground-wholemeal for preference. If these are not available use HiBran or wheatmeal or granary loaves
Biscuits	Ryvita, Mcvitie's, Crackawheat and similar varieties Digestive, oatcakes, coconut, and bran biscuits, etc.
Wholemeal flour or 100% rye flour	Should be used with white flour for making bread, scones, cakes, biscuits, puddings, etc.
Fresh fruit and vegetables	Should be used at least twice daily; the skin and peel of fruit and vegetables, apples, pears, plums, tomatoes and potatoes should be eaten
Dried fruit and nuts	Use frequently
Brown rice, wholemeal pasta	
Pulse vegetables	Such as peas and all varieties of beans

Artificial sweeteners (Table 8.3) containing aspartame or saccharin are free of both carbohydrate and calories. They are damaged by heat and should be added after cooking. Fructose and sorbitol are used in some proprietary foods; their calorie content is high and sorbitol can cause diarrhoea.

Proprietary 'diabetic foods' found in many supermarkets are usually

Table 8.3 Artificial sweeteners

Aspartame-based	Hermesetas Gold
	Canderel
	Sweetex Plus
Saccharin-based	Sweetex
	Saxin
	Hermesetas

Sugarlite, Sucron and Sweetex powders contain sugar and should not be used. Sorbitol and fructose are suitable for baking but high in calories

expensive and high in calorie content. They are not recommended although diabetic squash and 'diet' and low calorie fizzy drinks are suitable; special chocolate and marmalade are appreciated by many. Fruit juice, often labelled 'no added sugar' is not suitable for diabetics because of its high intrinsic sugar content; liberal use of such juices is frequently a hidden cause of poor control.

Alcohols containing simple sugar should not be used by diabetics, especially sweet wines and liqueurs. Dry wines and spirits are mainly sugar-free and do not present special problems. Beers and lagers have a relatively high sugar content and their amount needs to be both limited and counted as a part of the controlled carbohydrate intake. Sugar-free beers are high in calorie and alcohol content and have therefore some limitations to their usefulness. Profound hypoglycaemia may be provoked in those who take large amounts of alcohol, especially spirits, and omit their normal diet, especially in those taking sulphonylureas; this can be very dangerous. Normal social drinking is usually free from this hazard but care is still needed.

Special requirements for insulin-treated patients

If patients using insulin eat too little or omit meals, they become hypoglycaemic; if they eat too much at the wrong time they become hyperglycaemic. For optimal control, and particularly to avoid hypoglycaemia, much more finesse is needed in their dietary management. The important principles are that the carbohydrate intake should be steady from day to day and that it should be taken at fairly regular times of day. Carbohydrate restriction is not necessarily required, but a controlled amount is important.

Insulin-treated patients therefore must be able to calculate the carbohydrate content of their food, although weighing is not necessary. The actual carbohydrate content varies considerably from about 100 g daily for elderly or sedentary patients to 300 g (or occasionally more) for adolescent males and those with heavy manual occupations. Diets containing much more or much less carbohydrate than these limits may lead to problems with control.

For social convenience it is customary to advise that most of the carbohydrate is taken at main meals — breakfast, lunch and dinner. Snacks between meals are very important indeed for prevention of hypoglycaemia, especially those taken mid-morning and at bed-time when patients are particularly vulnerable to this problem. These snacks should never be missed.

For convenience 10 g of carbohydrate is described as 'one portion' so that a 150 g carbohydrate diet is described to patients as one of '15 portions'. Patients need to know the number of carbohydrate portions of different foodstuffs.

Table 8.4 A sample meal plan

	Carbohydrate portions	Recommended food and drink
Breakfast	1	Fruit
	1	Wholemeal cereal
	1	Milk
	1	Wholemeal bread
		Egg/grilled bacon
		Tea/coffee
Mid-morning	1	Fruit/plain biscuit
		Tea/coffee/diet drink
Lunch		Lean meat/fish/egg/cheese
	2	Potatoes/bread/rice/pasta
		Vegetable salad
	2	Fruit/sugar-free pudding
Mid-afternoon	1	Fruit/plain biscuit
		Tea/coffee/diet drink
Dinner		Lean meat/fish/eggs/cheese
	2	Potatoes/bread/rice/pasta
		Vegetable salad
	2	Fruit/sugar free pudding
Bed-time	1	Bread/fruit/plain biscuit
		Tea/coffee/diet drink
	Total 15	

The diets

Main recommendations centre round three main groupings: (1) foods which must be avoided (i.e. those containing simple sugars); (2) foods which may be taken freely; and (3) foods containing complex carbohydrates, which should be regulated.

FOODS TO AVOID

These foods contain sugar and inevitably upset the control of diabetes.

1 Confectionery and preserves: sugar, glucose, Sucron, jam, marmalade, honey, syrup, treacle, lemon curd, chocolate spread, all sweets, chocolates, fudge, toffee, mints, boiled sweets.

2 Sweet drinks: ordinary squash or fizzy drinks, e.g. Ribena, Lucozade, coke, tonic water, milkshakes (e.g. Nutrament, Complan), sweetened or unsweetened fruit juice.

3 Cakes and sweet biscuits: chocolate, filled or sweet biscuits, all sweet cakes, sweet pastries or pies.

4 Sweet puddings: fruit tinned in syrup, sweet ready made desserts, sweet sauces, sweetened condensed milk, mincemeat, fancy ice cream.

5 Sweet breakfast cereals: Frosties, Sugar Puffs, honey coated bran, sweetened muesli, Coco Pops, Ricicles, etc.

6 Alcohol: sweet wines, sherries, cider or liqueurs. Strong lagers (e.g. Tennants Extra, Red Stripe, Carlsberg Special Brew, Pils, Hemeling, etc.).

FOODS WHICH MAY BE TAKEN FREELY

These foods contain very little or no carbohydrate and do *not* affect diabetic control.

1 Drinks: clear soups, coffee, tea, soda water, low calorie or 'diet' drinks, diabetic squash, tomato juice, lemon juice, mineral water.

2 Vegetables: all green leafy vegetables, cauliflower, broccoli, onions, green beans, mushrooms, peppers, carrots, swedes, cho-cho, cucumber, celery, tomatoes, beansprouts, radish, ackee, karela, okra, endives, chicory, artichoke, mooli, calaloo, etc.

3 Fruits: berries and currants (not dried), e.g. gooseberries, strawberries, raspberries, red and blackcurrants, bitter fruits such as lemons, rhubarb, grapefruit and watermelon.

4 Seasonings: pepper, mustard, curry powder, herbs, spices, vinegar, Marmite, Bovril, Worcester sauce, stock cubes, etc.).

FOODS CONTAINING COMPLEX CARBOHYDRATES

These foods can and should be used by diabetic patients, but in regulated amounts since they do cause hyperglycaemia. In particular, insulin-treated patients should generally know their approximate carbohydrate content so

Table 8.5 A diet to lose weight

To lose weight, low-calorie, high-fibre carbohydrate foods should be used (e.g. wholemeal bread, pasta and cereal, fruit and vegetables) and fatty foods should be avoided. Patients should attempt not to exceed the following amounts:

Meat and fish
Maximum cooked portion of 3 oz (85 g) meat or 4 oz (110 g) fish
Visible fat should be removed; food should not be fried

Cheese
Hard cheese, e.g. cheddar, blue cheese: 4 oz (110 g)/week
Low fat cheese, e.g. Tendale, Shape: 6 oz (170 g)/week
Cottage cheese, curd cheese: any quantity

Eggs
Three per week, not fried

Milk
Low fat milks have the same amount of carbohydrate as ordinary milk, only the fat is removed
Whole milk: 1/2 pint (0.25 l)/day (fresh, dried or long-life)
Skimmed: 1 pint (0.5 l)/day

Fats
Avoid cooking with fat or eating any fried or greasy food
Any oils: very little per week
Butter, Flora, Krona, margarine: 4 oz (110 g)/week
Low-fat spread, e.g. Delight, Outline: 8 oz (225 g)/week

Alcohol
All alcohol is high in calories. Non-alcoholic, sugar-free drinks should be used

Sauces and dressings
Rich sauces and dressings should be avoided, e.g. mayonnaise, salad cream, French dressing. Lemon juice, natural yoghurt or vinegar can be used instead

Patients are also advised on regular exercise; they should weigh themselves weekly at the same time of day in the same clothes, and aim to lose about 1 lb (0.5 kg) a week.

---

that they can take the right amount at the right time (see p. 88). Food products are now often labelled with the carbohydrate and fat content. Helpful details are available in leaflets from several supermarket groups.

1 Bread: it is best to use wholemeal, granary, or high-bran, rolls or crispbread; chapati, naan bread and paratha are suitable if not too fatty.

2 Cereals: the best are wholegrain breakfast cereals such as Weetabix, branflakes, shredded wheat and porridge.

3 Rice and pasta: where possible, brown rice and wholemeal pasta should be used.

4 Potatoes: jacket, boiled or mashed potatoes are best. Chips and roast potatoes should be avoided.

Table 8.6 Simple sugars for use when treating hypoglycaemia

20–30 g of sugar is normally needed; the following each contain 10 g of sugar:

Lucozade	60 ml (4 tablespoons)
Ribena	15 ml (1 tablespoon)
	(to be diluted)
Coca-cola	90 ml
Sugar	2 teaspoons
Sugar lumps	3
Dextrosol tablets	3
Hypostop (glucose gel)	2

Foods suitable during intercurrent illness
For patients who are feeling ill but need to maintain their carbohydrate intake, the following are useful (each item contains 10 g (1 portion) of carbohydrate):
1/3 pint (0.15 l) tinned soup
1 glass fruit juice
1 scoop of ice cream
1 glass of milk

The following each contain 20 g of carbohydrate:
2 teaspoons Horlicks and milk
2 digestive biscuits
1 Weetabix and a glass of milk
1 ordinary fruit yoghurt
'Build-up' made with 1/2 pint (0.25 l) of milk and 1 sachet contains 40 g carbohydrate

5   Biscuits: wholemeal, plain or semi-sweet biscuits may be eaten, e.g. digestives, Krackerwheat, Ryvita, Rich Tea, Morning Coffee.
6   Milk: no more than 1 pint (1/2 litre) of milk per day. Skimmed or semi-skimmed milk is preferred.
7   Fruits: fruit intake should not usually exceed three helpings each day. Sugar-free stewed fruit or tinned fruit can be used.
8   Pulses: most beans and pulses may be taken freely, e.g. kidney beans, lentils, chick peas, etc. Baked beans in tomato sauce should be limited unless unsweetened.

Samples of diets for weight loss, a meal plan and suitable simple sugars for treating hypoglycaemia are shown in Tables 8.4–6.

Further reading

British Diabetic Association (1983). *Dietary Recommendations for Diabetics for the 1980s — a Policy Statement by the Nutrition Sub-committee.* London, British Diabetic Association
Hadden D.R. (1982). Food and diabetes: the dietary treatment of insulin dependent and non-insulin dependent diabetes. *Clinics in Endocrinology and Metabolism,* **11**, 503–524

9: Insulin Treatment

The discovery of insulin has been one of the major medical triumphs of the twentieth century. Even now, it is remarkable to witness the spectacular improvement in health and well-being which are experienced when insulin-dependent patients start treatment. Hypoglycaemia remains the single major hazard encountered in using insulin, feared by all those who take it, and insulin regimes must be devised to avoid this problem.

Insulin is needed for the treatment of all IDD patients, for many NIDD patients whose treatment with oral hypoglycaemic agents has failed, for all diabetics whose control deteriorates in the presence of intercurrent illness, and is usually essential in diabetic pregnancy. More details defining the criteria for starting insulin are given on p. 8 and in Table 9.1.

Many NIDD patients need insulin for well-being rather than for survival and a detailed description regarding the indications for insulin is given on p. 94. NIDD patients whose control worsens during intercurrent illness should usually be treated with insulin, while diabetic pregnant women should always be given insulin if diet alone has failed. Insulin is always needed after total pancreatectomy.

Table 9.1 Indications for insulin treatment

Symptoms	*Age*
Rapid onset	Any, more likely under 30
Substantial weight loss	
Weakness	*Other indications*
Vomiting	When tablets have failed
	During pregnancy when diet fails
Signs	During intercurrent illness
Usually thin	After pancreatectomy
Dry tongue	
Weak	*Any blood glucose concentration*
Ketoacidosis	
Drowsiness	
Dehydration	
Overbreathing	
Breath smelling of acetone	

Objectives of insulin treatment

When insulin treatment is started it is important to have clear aims for the individual patient. These will need to be one or more of the following:

1   For survival and prevention of ketoacidosis.
2   To alleviate symptoms.
3   To enable patients to live a full and active life.
4   To achieve good control and, if possible, prevent the development of long-term complications.

The first two aims are readily achieved with almost any insulin regime; some elderly patients or those who lack motivation can achieve no more. Most sensible patients who are well advised, will live almost normal lives with very few restrictions while taking insulin. The attainment of very good control is however much more difficult, and quite often causes unacceptable and dangerous episodes of hypoglycaemia; advice on this subject needs to be given by specialists who really understand the problems. Difficulties with 'control' and hypoglycaemia are the most frequent subjects of consultations at a diabetic clinic.

The insulins

Most patients in Western Europe are now using human insulins which have the same structure as that normally secreted in man. It is commercially prepared either by chemical manipulation of insulin extracted from the pancreas of pigs (enzymatically manipulated pork or 'emp') or by genetic manipulation of *Escherichia coli* (recombinant human insulin, 'crb' or 'prb'). The availability of beef insulin is decreasing, while porcine insulin is still widely available. All insulins in the UK are now at a single strength of 100 U/ml.

The purity of insulins now available is a striking tribute to developments since the earlier days of treatment in the 1920s when the huge volumes of impure fluid led to pain and major reactions at the sites of injection. Problems from insulin allergy, local skin reactions and insulin resistance have virtually disappeared. Insulin antibodies still develop even in patients taking pure human preparations, but titres are lower than previously and they apparently have no significant clinical effects.

Insulins are manufactured in four forms — as soluble insulin, isophane (protamine-linked) insulin, insulin zinc suspensions, and as ready-mixed combinations, of which there are increasing numbers. All the insulins are cloudy in appearance except for the soluble insulins which are clear.

Choice of the preferred combination and type of insulin preparation(s) for an individual patient is based on the duration of action; short-acting (soluble) and medium-acting insulins are used almost exclusively. The more

Table 9.2 Commonest available insulins in the UK

Soluble insulins	*Mixtures*
Human Actrapid*	Human Initard (50% velosulin, 50% insulatard)
Humulin S⁺	Human Mixtard (30% velosulin, 70% insulatard)
Human Velosulin* (also	(also porcine Mixtard and Initard)
porcine)	Human Actraphane (30% actrapid, 70% protophane)
	Humulin M1 (10% humulin S, 90% humulin I)
Isophane insulins	Humulin M2 (20% humulin S, 80% humulin I)
Human Insulatard* (also	Humulin M3 (30% humulin S, 70% humulin I)
porcine)	Humulin M4 (40% humulin S, 60% humulin I)
Humulin I⁺	
Human Protophane*	
Zinc suspensions	
Humulin Lente⁺	
Humulin Zn⁺	
Human Monotard*	
Human Ultratard*	

* Enzymatically manipulated pork (emp).
⁺ Biosynthetic human insulin (prb).
Bovine insulins are still available as Hypurin Neutral, Isophane, Lente and Protamine Zinc from CP Pharmaceuticals. Other insulins such as Rapitard, Lentard and Semitard are still available.

sustained duration of the only available truly long-acting insulin, Human Ultratard, has rather limited application. It is however important to observe that duration of any individual insulin varies considerably from one patient to another, and in practice can only be discovered by trial and error. Duration depends on many factors including dose, site of injection, presence of insulin antibodies, renal function and presumably other complex factors as well. Full details of available insulins are given in Table 9.2.

Short-acting (soluble) insulins

These are rapidly absorbed with onset of action within 0.5–1 hour, a peak action at about 3–4 hours, generally lasting no more than about 8 hours.

Intermediate insulins

These include isophane insulin and some of the insulin–zinc preparations. Isophane insulins include Insulatard, Humulin I and Protophane. Amorphous and crystalline zinc insulins confer longer or shorter durations of action on the preparation, and they are often provided in combinations. The most popular of the zinc insulin suspensions are Monotard and Humulin Zinc Insulin; Lentard and the shorter-acting Semitard are also available though probably less useful. Their duration of action is very variable, perhaps between 12 and 20 hours. Ready mixed insulins include mixtures of soluble and intermediate or long-acting insulins in different proportions.

Indications for insulin treatment

All patients with acute symptoms from IDD or ketoacidosis need insulin urgently (p. 96). Insulin treatment can be required at any age, even amongst the very old. Most, though not all, patients under thirty years of age will need insulin. The level of the blood glucose taken in isolation does not indicate the need for insulin, although most cases in which it exceeds 25 mmol/l are likely to need it. Ketonuria (as opposed to ketoacidosis) usually, but not always, suggests that insulin treatment is required: it is sometimes due to starvation.

Starting insulin treatment

The exact procedure depends on the individual circumstances; most patients are now started on insulin and managed entirely as out-patients. Only those who are ill from ketoacidosis or other causes, or incapable for reasons of age (young or old), physical defects (including vision) or personality problems require admission to hospital.

Out-patient management of insulin treatment requires the full team of doctors and specialist nurses, together with the availability of immediate telephone advice in the first few days. Patients are taught to give their own first injection which improves morale when they find it to be less unpleasant than expected. They usually learn to perform blood glucose monitoring and are given simple dietary advice. The major aim at this stage is to reduce hyperglycaemia without causing symptomatic hypoglycaemia which can shatter confidence if it occurs in the early days.

It is a mistake to attempt to teach too much immediately after diagnosis. Retention of information is poor and a more structured series of interviews with dietiticians and specialist nurses should follow during the next few days and weeks. Topics that need to be covered are shown in Table 9.3.

The regime needed at the start of insulin treatment depends on the circumstances: namely whether the patient is acutely ill; ambulant but acutely isulin-dependent; or whether the need for insulin has arisen more gradually in patients where oral hypoglycaemic agents have failed.

ACUTELY ILL PATIENTS

The treatment of patients who are severely ill and dehydrated requires intravenous insulin and fluids and is described on p. 96. Otherwise, in those who are less seriously ill, a soluble insulin preparation is used

Table 9.3 Topics to be covered on starting insulin

Days 1 and 2	Days 3 and 4
What is diabetes? (if new diabetic)	Check days 1 and 2
Importance of regular clinic attendance	
	Equipment
Insulin	Plastic syringe
Which?	Storage
When?	Insulin
Effect of insulin on blood glucose	Expiry date
Timing	
Dose	*Other syringes*
Drawing up	Glass
Sites and rotation	Fixed
Injecting at 90°	Click/count
	Novopen
Insulin card	
Relative taught	*Blood glucose testing*
	Type
Hypoglycaemia	Storage
Signs and symptoms	Technique
Treatment	Recording results
Dextrosol and carbohydrate	Interpretation
Recovery	Action
Causes	Profile
Glucagon	Exercise
Check	*Exercise*
Driving	What form?
Starter pack	Advice given
Telephone contact	
District Nurse	*Assessment*
Dietician	Competent?
	Needs to be re-checked

subcutaneously and is given three times daily. The daily starting dose may be between 20 and 30 units and should be adjusted each day. A sliding scale is of no value and should not be used. As the patient recovers the definitive long-term insulin regimen is instituted. For further details see p. 80.

AMBULANT INSULIN-DEPENDENT PATIENTS

Most newly-diagnosed IDD patients can start their treatment on an out-patient basis. A soluble insulin preparation given subcutaneously two or three times daily is needed in order to lower the blood glucose fairly quickly and eliminate symptoms. Some patients will start with a twice-daily mixture of soluble and medium-acting insulins, and some with medium-acting insulin alone. In the long-term, most patients will be treated with a regular mixture of soluble and medium-acting insulins (see below). For many, the ready mixed insulins will be more appropriate (Table 9.2). A safe starting dose for adult out-patients is between 10 and 20 units daily; accurate prediction of needs is not possible.

NIDD PATIENTS NEEDING INSULIN

These patients will respond well to most insulin regimes. They can be started using similar techniques to those described above. The use of ready-mixed insulins in this group is often appropriate and they may be used at the outset. Many, though not all, older patients will respond well to a single daily insulin injection.

Adjustment of insulin dose

When insulin has been started as an in-patient, achieving satisfactory control of blood glucose levels, it is essential to reduce the dose before leaving hospital, since the increased activity is certain to cause hypoglycaemia. The dose will need to be reduced by as much as 20–30% and then reviewed when the patient is back to normal activity.

The 'honeymoon'

Soon after starting insulin, many IDD patients experience a decrease in the insulin requirement, and may even be able to stop insulin altogether. This is described as the 'honeymoon' period. It occurs because of residual endogenous insulin secretion which persists for a few weeks or months. As the remaining insulin secretion declines, the patient's need for injected insulin increases. While it is sometimes possible for patients to manage without insulin for short periods, this practice is not normally recommended because of the great disappointment when insulin is inevitably restarted.

Long-term management

The needs of the long-term programme of treatment are as follows:
1 Maintenance of satisfactory blood glucose levels without symptomatic hypoglycaemia.
2 Appropriate dietary advice, compatible with the patient's body weight, lifestyle and insulin regime.
3 Continuing education to enable patients to make appropriate adjustments to insulin doses and diet both under normal circumstances and when intercurrent illness or other emergencies arise.

Insulin regimens

Most patients with IDD are managed with twice-daily insulin injections; once-daily insulin is rarely if ever satisfactory. Soluble and intermediate insulins are given together initially, with two-thirds of the total dose given in the morning, and with the intermediate insulin comprising two-thirds of each dose. Subsequent adjustments can then be made on the basis of home blood glucose monitoring and may eventually be very different from the starting regime (Fig. 9.1).

Overnight hypoglycaemia and unacceptable morning hyperglycaemia are common on this regimen. Improvement is often obtained by dividing the evening insulin dose so that soluble insulin alone is given before dinner, and the intermediate acting insulin at bed-time; this three-dose regime is very satisfactory for many patients.

An increasing number of patients now prefer taking four doses daily, chiefly because of the greater flexibility of lifestyle which results. Soluble insulin is given before each meal and a longer-acting preparation at bed-time. The three pre-meal doses are most easily given with one of the new 'pen devices' which meter the insulin dose which is delivered from an

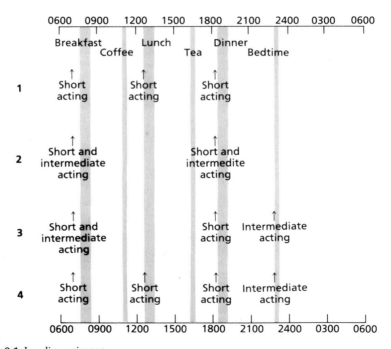

Fig. 9.1 Insulin regimens.

insulin cartridge (see p. 232). The device is easily carried without the need for spare syringes and needles.

The simplest regime is a single daily dose of insulin given before breakfast. This is suitable for many NIDD patients, and for some elderly patients who come to need insulin. Many will now use one of the ready-mixed insulins (e.g. Mixtard). There can be less trouble from nocturnal hypoglycaemia on this regime.

Technique of insulin treatment

Detailed advice regarding the technique of insulin administration is vital for well being and to achieve good control.

Equipment (see Appendix)

Disposable plastic syringes, usually with needle attached and now available on prescription are preferred by most patients; they can be re-used, and kept in a refrigerator between injections. Some long-established patients still prefer the old glass syringes. Pre-set glass syringes which deliver a fixed but adjustable amount of insulin are valuable for those with poor sight or those who find the technique difficult to learn. Click–count syringes help some blind patients, although the new 'pen' devices which deliver insulin in metered doses from an insulin cartridge should prove much better.

Sites and technique of insulin injection

Subcutaneous insulin is usually injected on the front of the thigh or into the abdominal wall; some patients prefer upper arms or buttocks. Sites should be rotated on a systematic basis in order to avoid fat hypertrophy and erratic insulin absorption which leads to unpredictable swings of blood glucose. Insulin absorption is more rapid from the abdomen and the arm than thigh or buttocks, and such variations occasionally underly difficulties with control.

Insulin should be injected into the subcutaneous tissue with the skin stretched between thumb and forefinger; the needle is inserted briskly at almost 90^0 to the skin, to almost its whole length. Cleaning with spirit and pulling back syringe plunger are not usually necessary. When the needle is withdrawn the injection site is pressed firmly with cotton wool.

Continuous subcutaneous infusion (CSII)

The concept of infusing insulin continuously with pre-prandial boosts, thus mimicking the action of the pancreas, was developed into the technique of

CSII at Guy's Hospital (see Appendix). CSII now has an established if limited role in the management of diabetes. Its principal indications are to improve the lifestyle of patients needing great flexibility, to alleviate the problems of recurring hypoglycaemia, and to achieve a very tight control, especially in pregnancy and painful neuropathy. Since most of these aims can now be achieved by other techniques of insulin administration, CSII is rarely used, but it can be outstandingly successful, and some patients are not easily parted from their pumps.

Soluble insulin is used in a syringe or in cartridge form, and driven continuously by a small pump feeding insulin through a fine cannula attached to a 25 or 27 g metal needle with wings which is inserted subcutaneously into the abdomen, and moved on alternate days. Initially half the usual daily dose is given as the basal infusion over 24 hours and the other half divided into three equal parts given 15–45 minutes before each of the three main meals.

Patients using CSII must be highly motivated, undertake regular blood glucose monitoring and be able to get expert advice throughout 24 hours. The technique is expensive and running costs are high. Mechanical failures, sepsis at infusion sites and weight gain are some of the problems encountered by patients. The greatest hazard is the very rapid development of severe ketoacidosis if the pump fails; patients should at all times have a conventional syringe and insulin available in case this occurs.

Insulin dose

Insulin doses cannot be predicted, and newly-diagnosed patients and those converted to insulin should be started very cautiously, unless they are ill or ketotic (see p. 102). The average dose for established IDD patients is 0.7 U/kg/day, but there is a wide range.

It is very important to remember that the dose of insulin gives no indication of the need for insulin; some patients are absolutely dependent for life on only a few units daily, while others (NIDD patients) who have been given very large amounts may manage satisfactorily with oral hypoglycaemic agents.

Monitoring treatment

All insulin-dependent patients should be encouraged to undertake blood glucose monitoring (see Chapter 7), although some patients are unable or unwilling to do so, and prefer urinalysis. A balance needs to be established between adequate documentation of control and excessive and obsessional introspection which home testing sometimes engenders. For most patients,

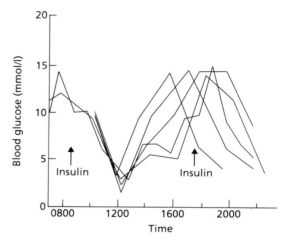

Fig. 9.2 Blood glucose profiles from a patient taking twice daily insulin injections.

an average of a single daily blood glucose measurement should suffice; if this is done at different times (Fig. 9.2) an overall pattern may be built up. In this way the peaks and troughs of blood glucose are discovered allowing intelligent changes of insulin dose, type and diet to be made.

Multiple daily profiles should be reserved for limited periods such as pregnancy, illness, or when the insulin regime is changed. Patients should never change the insulin dose on a daily basis, nor in response to single aberrant readings. Blood glucose measurement at bed-time is a most valuable practice which saves many patients, both adults and children, from developing nocturnal hypoglycaemia; if the level is less than 5 mmol/l, extra carbohydrate is taken. It is also particularly valuable before driving for the same reason. Measurement of blood glucose by parents or other relatives during an episode of unconsciousness helps to identify whether or not it is due to hypoglycaemia.

Most patients should aim for the peaks of blood glucose to be no higher than 10 mmol/l and the troughs not less than 4 mmol/l. Such are the vagaries of diabetes control, however, that it is inevitable that some readings will be higher, and others lower than these levels; this must be properly explained and patients taught not to panic.

A few patients become obsessed by blood glucose monitoring which comes to dominate their lives. This arises particularly in those who fail to understand the blood glucose profile and the need to detect peaks and troughs before changing their treatment. These patients undertake an increasing number of blood glucose estimations, change their insulin too often, and suffer multiple hypoglycaemic episodes. They often fear the development of complications even when single readings exceed normal. The frenzy which this causes is sometimes induced by doctors whose own experience is limited. Considerable patience and retraining is needed to reverse this unfortunate situation. A grateful patient wrote this letter: 'I was particularly interested by your comments about diabetic patients doing too many blood tests, resulting in neurotic patients. This was certainly true about me. I have passed this tip on to a diabetic friend who agreed that she had been reacting likewise — doing extra "jabs" when high blood sugars were recorded resulting in a hypo more often than not.'

Adjusting the insulin dose

Changes of insulin dose on any one day should normally be kept within 10–20% of the existing daily dose. Changes should not normally be made more than twice weekly. A common error in the adjustment of insulin is to alter the insulin dose immediately *after* a blood glucose reading instead of adjusting the *preceding* dose; this practice inevitably causes further instability.

When consistent daily fluctuations of blood glucose have been shown treatment should be modified, aiming chiefly to eliminate hypoglycaemic episodes and thereafter to obtain better control by increasing the blood glucose in the troughs and decreasing it at the peaks. Awareness of the duration of action of each insulin used is essential — a common problem is the use of too much short-acting and insufficient intermediate-acting insulin. The aim should be to obtain a smooth pattern without 'peaks and troughs'.

TO INCREASE BLOOD GLUCOSE

1 Reduce the dose of the appropriate insulin *before* the trough (e.g. decrease short-acting insulin if blood glucose is low before noon)
2 Eat more carbohydrate at or before the times when blood glucose values are at their lowest; the exact amount of extra carbohydrate can be determined only by trial and error.

TO DECREASE BLOOD GLUCOSE

1 Reduce by a little the amount of carbohydrate taken at the meals which precede the peaks by 2 or 3 hours.
2 Increase the dose of insulin *before* the peak.
      Soluble insulin should be altered to change blood glucose concentration within 2–6 hours and medium-acting insulin should be altered to change

blood glucose in 6–12 hours. The duration of insulin action varies considerably, however, and these figures provide only a rough guide.

Severely unstable ('brittle') diabetes

It is doubtful whether there is a true entity of 'brittle diabetes', and it has been said that there are only 'brittle diabetics'. The blood glucose profile of some patients may however show extreme swings, but this does not normally disrupt their lifestyle unless they become obsessed by the blood glucose readings themselves (p. 84). The lives of a few patients are, however, severely disrupted by frequent admissions to hospital, either due to hypoglycaemic or ketoacidotic causes. This situation is commonest in teenage girls; it is usually temporary and, as they mature, the problems vanish when life itself stabilizes with the security of employment and family life. There are several causes for such severe disruption of diabetes, ranging from simple technical errors, to gross deceptions of great ingenuity. Unravelling these problems requires patience and skill; technical errors must be identified, proper treatment advised, and social and psychological factors which might cause patients to be manipulative must be sought.

TECHNICAL ERRORS

Injection technique, faulty equipment, the wrong insulin and inability to see properly may all cause problems with diabetic control. In addition, incorrect blood and urine tests can lead to inappropriate adjustments to treatment. Failure to keep a proper dietary regime is a further obstacle to success.

MENSTRUATION

Diabetic control often changes in the pre-menstrual phase, usually requiring an increase of insulin dose. This rarely causes problems, but just occasionally the changes are sufficiently severe to cause monthly ketoacidosis. With careful planning the problem can usually be overcome.

PANCREATECTOMY

Blood glucose fluctuations after pancreatectomy can be very difficult to control. These patients require very small amounts of insulin, and minute changes of dose can have a disproportionate effect on blood glucose levels.

MANIPULATION OF DIABETES

If there is no demonstrable cause for disruptive diabetes, the patient needs hospital admission for observation. The problem is sometimes solved if the nursing staff take over insulin injections; if the problem returns when the patient resumes treatment, some form of manipulation is almost certain. Discovering the technique of manipulation is sometimes very difficult, and the true source of disruption may never be known; a hint by the physician that he knows of the deceit is sometimes curative, without causing the anger and aggression which result from an outright accusation, although sometimes that becomes necessary.

Considerable ingenuity can be employed in manipulating diabetes. Some patients give additional insulin, hidden in transistors, taped behind doors or windows or in the bottom of a jewel case. One patient was eventually found to drive the insulin needle into the skin and out again before depressing the plunger. Hypoglycaemia 2 days after 'stopping' insulin is an important clue, while application of glucose to the skin before blood glucose measurement causes absurd readings, with inappropriate treatment as a result. Falsified blood glucose and urine testing results are not rare and must be suspected if they are quite incompatible with the clinical problem.

Deep-seated emotional, social or psychiatric problems underly manipulation of diabetes. Discovering the exact cause is never easy. The problem can sometimes be reduced by patient support of the family, but on other occasions more formal family counselling is required. The advice of a psychiatrist should only be sought if there is real evidence of a psychiatric disorder. Very occasionally, patients are incapable of an independent life and may need institutional supervision.

Some years after manipulating her diabetes, a patient wrote this letter: 'At one clinic of yours which I attended you asked me if I was taking overdoses. I was stupid and did not admit this until December, 1981. I am still not as well balanced as I would like but I am better than I was.'

Management of diabetes during illness

During most illnesses or infections the blood glucose concentration tends to increase and diabetic control deteriorates. Most diabetics then need a larger dose of insulin than usual and some who normally take tablets come to need insulin. The increased need for insulin occurs even when patients stop eating or vomiting begins, because hepatic gluconeogenesis and therefore hyperglycaemia are stimulated by insulin lack.

When diabetics develop an illness their normal insulin dose should be continued, carbohydrate taken in some palatable fluid form and regular monitoring up to four times daily should be undertaken. If blood glucose readings persistently exceed 15 mmol/l the soluble insulin should be increased by approximately 4 units. Additional doses can be given at noon or bedtime (4–8 units). If vomiting continues without remission for more than a few hours admission to hospital for treatment with intravenous fluids and insulin is advisable to prevent ketoacidosis.

This aspect of diabetic management is often poorly understood by both patients and many doctors too. Continuing education is important because for some patients events of this kind may only occur once or twice during the diabetic lifetime. It is helpful to give every insulin treated diabetic a small printed card with the simple instruction that insulin should never be stopped, together with other details describing exactly how to proceed in case of an emergency. These instructions should include a telephone number so that further advice can be obtained from a member of the diabetic team.

Stopping insulin

Insulin should not normally be stopped; withdrawal of insulin, even when no food is taken, leads to a rapid increase in hepatic gluconeogenesis and hyperglycaemia results often with the subsequent development of ketoacidosis as well.

Occasionally, in NIDD patients when insulin has been started during intercurrent illness, insulin can be withdrawn after recovery. Patients whose diabetes developed in 'hyperosmolar aketotic coma' (p. 104) can sometimes, but not always, be treated eventually with oral hypoglycaemic agents. Withdrawal of insulin should always be undertaken under strict supervision with gradual reduction of the dose; admission to hospital is sometimes advisable. If control with insulin is inadequate, withdrawal of insulin usually fails. The transition from insulin to tablets is sometimes helped by overlapping these treatments for about 2 days.

Changing insulin species

When patients are changed from beef to human insulin, an overall reduction of insulin dose of about 20% in the first instance is needed if insulin doses are over approximately 50 units daily, otherwise severe hypoglycaemia may occur. Thereafter, the dose is adjusted according to blood glucose levels. No dose change is needed when converting from porcine to human insulin, though some patients claim that they lose hypoglycaemic awareness after the change.

Diet for insulin-treated patients

Regular amounts of carbohydrate at regular times of day are important in insulin-treated patients in order to minimize swings of blood glucose, and in particular to avoid hypoglycaemia (Chapter 8). There is no technique

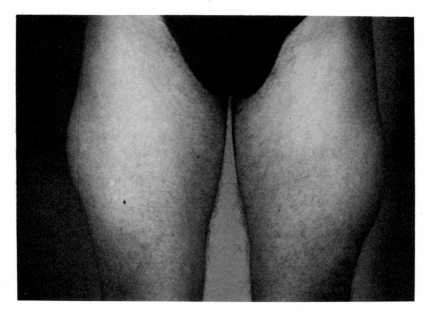

Fig. 9.3 Fat hypertrophy of overused sites of insulin injection.

of insulin administration which mimics the almost instantaneous release of pancreatic insulin following a meal; even the shortest-acting insulins injected subcutaneously have residual hypoglycaemic effects extending beyond 6 hours. The importance of snacks mid-morning, mid-afternoon and at bed-time between breakfast, lunch and dinner are therefore of critical importance to avoid hypoglycaemia. This is relatively simple for those who work regular hours and cook for themselves, but more difficult for those whose lifestyle is erratic or when others cater for their meals.

Problems associated with insulin injections

Blurring of vision is common during the first few days after starting insulin; reading becomes difficult, and unless this is explained to patients they may be very worried. It is due to changes of refraction, and corrects itself after about 3 weeks.

Oedema of the feet also occurs sometimes during the first 2 or 3 weeks of insulin treatment. It is always transient, and rarely requires treatment with diuretics.

Problems at the injection sites have decreased considerably with increasing purity of insulins; nevertheless, injection sites should be inspected regularly. The commonest defect now seen is fat hypertrophy; these fatty lumps develop at injection sites especially if a small area is used too frequently (Fig. 9.3). The fatty tumours may cause faulty and erratic absorption of insulin, leading sometimes to difficulties with diabetic control. Occasionally they are so disfiguring that excision is required. The best advice to patients is to rotate sites of insulin injection in a systematic pattern. Fat atrophy, previously common in women, is now rarely seen. Even the itchy red marks occurring during the first few weeks of insulin treatment are now uncommon, and abscesses at injection sites are remarkably rare. A few patients inadvertently give their insulin intradermally by injecting horizontally; such injections are painful and cause severe scarring.

Insulin allergy causing generalized urticaria is now outstandingly rare, although it has been reported even with human insulin; desensitization may be needed in such a case.

Insulin resistance

This has become very uncommon as insulin purity has increased. It may be defined as the need for more than 200 units of insulin daily for more than 1 week in the absence of obvious precipitating factors (e.g. pregnancy, steroids). It is usually seen when overweight patients are given insulin inappropriately, and it occasionally occurs when patients restart insulin having taken it months or years before. Insulin receptor defects, sometimes associated with acanthosis nigricans cause severe insulin resistance, but are very rare (p. 25).

Some cases of insulin resistance can be overcome by high rates of IV insulin infusion; intraperitoneal insulin has also been used in some instances.

Future developments

Alternatives to insulin injection would be desirable but have so far been unsuccessful. Oral insulin fails because it is rapidly degraded by gut enzymes, and membrane encapsulated insulin has not yet become a useful technique. Buccal and intranasal routes of insulin administration may succeed in theory but are inadequate in practice. The concept of an implantable 'artificial pancreas' is the subject of intensive research; an implantable glucose sensor is an essential part of such a device, and impressive advances are in progress at the present time. Intraperitoneal insulin delivery, which mimics the natural route of delivery and allows a first-pass effect of insulin on the liver has its advocates, and the use of gas-driven implantable pumps has had a limited success.

Insulin analogues and proinsulin can now be synthesized; with differential effects on hepatic and peripheral glucose disposal, or with advantageous durations of action, they may come to have a special role.

These insulins are still under development and clinical trial.

Pancreatic or islet transplantation might provide the ideal solution to diabetes treatment if they could be achieved without harming the patient. Pancreatic transplantation is technically feasible but is a major undertaking, and requires immunosuppression; it is usually done in association with a renal transplant, and is unethical at other times. Fewer than half the pancreatic transplants continue to function for more than 1 year, but when they are successful, they can transform the life of the patient and this may be sufficient justification in itself. The concept of islet transplantation is very appealing, but only partial successes have been obtained and suitable techniques are not yet available for use in man.

Further reading

Tattersall R.B. (1986). *Diabetes: a Practical Guide for Patients on Insulin*, 2nd edn. Churchill Livingstone, Edinburgh

10: Treatment of Non-Insulin-Dependent Diabetes

Three measures are available for treatment of NIDD, namely diet, oral hypoglycaemic agents and insulin. Diet, and especially the control of obesity, is the cornerstone of treatment. The more intensive and appropriate the advice, the less the need for the addition of tablet treatment which should, in any case, never be used as a substitute for failure to keep to the right diet. Dietary management is discussed in Chapter 8.

Treatment for patients with impaired glucose tolerance (IGT) only is discretionary. In general, younger patients, who are likely to become frankly diabetic, are treated by diet, especially if they are overweight, and kept under review. Older patients may be asked to lose weight if that is appropriate but can be discharged. If IGT occurs in pregnancy, patients are treated as if they were diabetic (Chapter 18).

Oral hypoglycaemic agents

Tablets should be prescribed when the physician is satisfied that dietary measures alone have failed. Sulphonylureas are generally preferred to biguanides because they are more effective and have fewer side effects. Biguanides are often used as the first treatment in grossly obese patients, but their use is otherwise mainly confined to those patients in whom sulphonylureas have failed. Doses should be kept to a minimum and attempts made to withdraw or reduce medication whenever possible.

About 30% of all diabetics use oral hypoglycaemic drugs. They should not generally be used during pregnancy although they are not known to be teratogenic. There are some restrictions on their use, especially in patients with renal impairment.

Sulphonylureas

Sulphonamides were observed to cause hypoglycaemia during their early development in the 1940s and sulphonylureas were developed in France as a direct result of this observation. Tolbutamide and chlorpropamide were introduced into clinical practice in 1956 and 1957 respectively and, although many others have been manufactured since then, there have been no major advances as a result. Sulphonylureas act chiefly by stimulating insulin

91

Table 10.1 Oral hypoglycaemic agents

Drug	Dose range (mg/day)
Sulphonylureas	
Glibenclamide	2.5–15
Glipizide	2.5–40
Gliclazide	40–320
Tolbutamide	500–2000
Chlorpropamide	100–500
Tolazamide	100–750
Gliquidone	15–180
Glibornuride	12.5–75
Acetohexamide	500–1500
Glymidine	500–2000
Biguanide	
Metformin	1000–3000

release from the islet B-cells together with some additional peripheral effects in lowering blood glucose as well. They are of no value in patients with IDD, whose islets have ceased to function, and of no particular advantage in patients with NIDD who come to need insulin. Since sulphonylureas stimulate insulin release, they also stimulate weight gain. They are therefore undesirable in the presence of obesity unless dietary treatment has failed and significant symptoms persist.

There are nine sulphonylureas and glymidine which is a sulpha-pyrimidine. They are remarkably safe and free from side effects, although rashes and more rarely still jaundice have been reported. Only one sulphonylurea should be used at a time since there is little evidence that they differ in potency and no benefit from combining more than one.

Hypoglycaemia is the chief hazard of sulphonylureas; it may be prolonged and even fatal but, considering the extensive use of these drugs, it is relatively uncommon and very rare if they are used correctly. The danger of hypoglycaemia exists chiefly in the elderly and in those with renal impairment; it occurs mainly when the longer-acting preparations such as chlorpropamide (half-life 36 hours) or glibenclamide (half-life 8 hours) are used. Selection of a sulphonylurea should therefore take these factors into account. Chlorpropamide is best avoided altogether and glibenclamide should not generally be used in old people or those in renal failure. Agents such as gliclazide or tolbutamide are more appropriate in these circumstances and are predominantly metabolized before being excreted.

Many diabetics taking chlorpropamide experience an unpleasant facial burning and flushing very shortly after drinking even small amounts of alcohol — the 'chlorpropamide-alcohol flush'. This does not generally occur with other sulphonylurea preparations and, if it does, the drug should be changed. This side effect is another reason to avoid the use of chlorpropamide.

Chlorpropamide also has an interesting effect of sensitizing the renal tubules to the actions of endogenous vasopressin; it is thus of use in partial pituitary diabetes insipidus and, on very rare occasions, in diabetics, it has been reported as a cause of hyponatraemia.

DRUG INTERACTIONS

These are uncommon. Alcohol can potentiate the action of sulphonylureas and the combination can be dangerous. Aspirin, sulphonamides and monoamine oxidase inhibitors may enhance their hypoglycaemic action, but the danger is relatively small and these drugs should be used if they are needed. Corticosteroids exacerbate hyperglycaemia, sometimes seriously if doses are high, and patients may need to be changed to insulin. The hyperglycaemic action of thiazides is usually mild though there are exceptions and they are best avoided; loop diuretics are less of a problem. Oral contraceptives have a negligible effect on control.

Biguanides

The hypoglycaemic action of these drugs was reported in 1957; they reduce hepatic gluconeogenesis, increase peripheral uptake of glucose and also to some extent reduce the absorption of carbohydrates. They do not require intact islets in order to exert their effect but even so are of no practical value in insulin-treated patients.

Metformin is the only biguanide which should be used because others, notably phenformin may, albeit rarely, cause lactic acidosis. This has been reported with metformin in patients with renal failure or any state of shock, and it should not be used in those patients, in the elderly or in those with liver disease.

Metformin has several unpleasant side effects which include nausea, diarrhoea and sometimes vomiting, which may be transient, and it may cause a disagreeable metallic taste in the mouth. Some patients suffer an insidious malaise and are grateful when the drug is withdrawn. Malabsorption syndromes have been reported. Some patients undergo extensive investigations for diarrhoea which subsequently ceases when metformin is stopped.

Guar gum

The presence of very high fibre content in food reduces the absorption of carbohydrate and thereby may reduce hyperglycaemia. The clinical effect of guar gum preparations is however very limited; a large dose is needed before each meal and the flatulence which they induce, though decreasing with use, is often intolerable. There are several preparations (e.g. Glucotard, Guarem, Guarina, Lejguar) but their role in the management of diabetes is very small.

Glucosidase inhibitors

Agents acting as enzyme inhibitors can reduce the breakdown of complex carbohydrates and thereby reduce their absorption. They effectively reduce the increase in blood glucose after a meal; they also cause flatulence. Their role in the treatment of NIDD is still being evaluated.

Insulin

The decision to start insulin treatment in an NIDD patient is not an easy one, especially amongst the many older diabetics who are overweight and poorly controlled. Many considerations are needed, as follows:

1 Ensure as far as possible that the recommended diet is kept, that oral hypoglycaemics are being taken, and that medications which exacerbate hyperglycaemia (e.g. thiazide diuretics) are stopped. These aspects require intensive care and education, and a home visit can be invaluable. Sometimes admission to hospital achieves all these aims and demonstrates to the patients that good control can be achieved.

2 If the weight is decreasing, patients are likely to need insulin; if it is increasing, they are more likely to be over-eating.

3 If diabetic symptoms persist on maximal oral therapy, a patient is likely to need insulin.

4 Some patients just manage to maintain adequate control by exceptionally rigorous dieting; tell-tale signs are a lean patient, often still losing weight, whose urine tests show evidence of ketonuria. Insulin treatment with an adequate diet has a miraculous effect on such a patient.

5 Poorly controlled, overweight patients who deny symptoms present a serious dilemma. If one is satisfied that they are keeping to their prescribed treatment (and frequently they are not) then insulin should probably be tried; insulin resistance and further weight gain are common problems in this situation. There are times therefore when insulin treatment for these patients is just not appropriate.

6 The development of early diabetic complications or hyperlipidaemia strengthens the decision to tighten control by starting insulin treatment.

7 The denial of symptoms should not deter the physician from recommending insulin treatment; most patients feel better after the change, even when symptoms were not apparent.

It is sometimes difficult to persuade these patients to take insulin. A very practical arrangement whereby insulin is recommended as a trial for 1 month in the first instance can help; most patients feel the benefit and opt to continue. If they do not improve, nothing has been lost and oral hypoglycaemics can be resumed.

Insulin regimes are considered in Chapter 9. A NIDD patient needing insulin is more likely than an IDD patient to be satisfactorily treated with a single daily injection.

Other indications for insulin in NIDD patients

When NIDD patients are under the stress of intercurrent illness, or pregnancy, insulin may be needed temporarily. Thus, many patients require insulin if they develop an infection or almost any medical emergency. Special vigilance is needed at the time of surgery (p. 109). If urinary tract infection is severe, elimination of glycosuria by insulin treatment can be important to stem the multiplication of the organisms.

If pregnancy is planned, insulin treatment is recommended. Once patients are pregnant, insulin should be used rather than tablets.

Further reading

Multi-Centre Study (1983). UK prospective study of therapies of maturity-onset diabetes. I. effect of diet, sulphonylureas, insulin or biguanide therapy on fasting plasma glucose and body weight over one year. *Diabetologia*, **24**, 404–411

11: Diabetic Emergencies: Ketoacidosis, Hypoglycaemia and Management during Surgery

Diabetic ketoacidosis

Ketoacidosis results from lack of insulin. It is a critical medical emergency requiring urgent hospital admission for administration of intravenous fluids and insulin. It should be avoidable. In practice, the chief causes, in order of frequency are:

1 Omission or reduction of insulin.
2 Undiagnosed diabetes.
3 Intercurrent illness, especially acute infections.
4 Unknown.

Biochemistry (Fig. 11.1)

The biochemical upset in severe diabetic ketoacidosis is very great. The

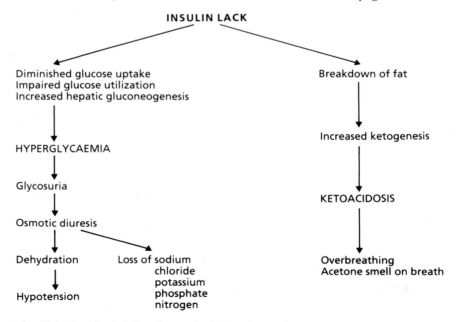

Fig. 11.1 Physiological disturbances in diabetic ketoacidosis.

prime fault is the lack of insulin which leads to a diminished uptake and utilization of glucose by the tissues, increased glucose formation from protein, and breakdown of fat in the liver and in adipose tissue. At the same time there is an increased secretion of stress hormones notably glucagon but also cortisol, catecholamines and growth hormone. Glucagon in particular accelerates the rise in glucose and ketogenesis at a time of insulin lack. The result of these major changes is a rise in the blood levels of glucose, non-esterified fatty acids and ketone bodies, chiefly acetoacetate and β-hydroxybutyrate (and also acetone). Increased glucose levels result in an osmotic diuresis, dehydration, loss of electrolytes and in severe cases to peripheral circulatory failure. Increased ketone levels lead to acidosis, vomiting, further loss of electrolytes and further dehydration from the overbreathing produced by the fall in pH.

The extent of the loss of water, electrolytes and nitrogen has been determined clinically by balance studies in which the amounts of these constituents retained by patients recovering from diabetic ketoacidosis were measured. The losses are considerable (Table 11.1).

Table 11.1 Average water and electrolyte losses in ketoacidosis

Water	6 litres
Sodium	500 mmol
Potassium	350 mmol
Chloride	400 mmol

Mortality

Before the introduction of insulin many diabetics eventually died from ketoacidosis and some still do. The condition is however preventable and this should not occur. Every case of ketoacidosis is the fault of someone — patient, parent, practitioner or physician. Nevertheless episodes of severe diabetic ketoacidosis are still common in clinical practice. Most cases occur in younger patients, but no patient and no age is immune.

There is still an average mortality of 9% for ketoacidosis. Though most deaths occur in older patients, usually from other major disorders from which they suffer, a small number of deaths still occur at all ages from avoidable causes. These are particularly the inhalation of gastric contents if no nasogastric tube has been inserted in those whose consciousness is obtunded, and hypokalaemia if proper monitoring is not carried out during treatment.

Causes of ketoacidosis

REDUCTION OF INSULIN

This is the quickest way of developing ketoacidosis. The patient on insulin should be told never to stop or reduce it during illness. In practice, insulin may be stopped inadvertently, as a result of bad advice or wilfully.

UNDIAGNOSED DIABETES

About one-quarter of all cases of ketoacidosis occurs in previously undi-agnosed diabetics. However diabetic ketoacidosis never develops suddenly and symptoms have invariably been present usually for weeks or months, although their significance may have been missed. It is still unfortunately fairly common for patients to complain to their doctors of thirst, polyuria and loss of weight and for their blood or urine glucose not to be tested. The diagnosis of diabetes is still often missed although it should be easy (see p. 9).

INTERCURRENT ILLNESS, ESPECIALLY ACUTE INFECTION

Intercurrent illnesses, especially if accompanied by vomiting, usually increase the need for insulin; those on tablets may require insulin while they are ill. Infections, commonly urinary or chest infections, are most often the culprits. It is disastrous to stop or even reduce the dose of insulin at this time and, even if the normal dose is maintained in these situations, that may not be sufficient to prevent ketoacidosis. Details of managing diabetes during intercurrent illness are given on p. 86.

UNIDENTIFIED CAUSES

Diabetic ketoacidosis may develop for no obvious reason; in some patients who are apparently well stabilized the need for insulin may rapidly increase for no known reason and the patient or his doctor may not be quick enough to realize what is happening. Insulin resistance can occur pre-menstrually and lead to ketoacidosis. As with intercurrent infections, if a diabetic starts to vomit, this frequently hastens the development of ketoacidosis. Vomiting in an insulin-requiring diabetic always requires vigilance.

Most diabetics never have an episode of ketoacidosis. This is because they are sensible and have been well taught how to manage their diabetes, particularly in the presence of intercurrent illness. There are unfortunately a few patients, usually girls in their teens, who repeatedly develop keto-acidosis, perhaps as a result of manipulating their diabetes. This serious although uncommon problem is described in more detail on p. 86.

Clinical features

Ketoacidosis never develops suddenly. Symptoms characteristic of uncontrolled diabetes (notably thirst and polyuria) appear over several days or sometimes longer, though occasionally and especially in the young the cause of the illness evolves over a few hours. The osmotic diuresis causes increasing fluid loss and, as dehydration progresses, vomiting begins, and exacerbates the situation. If symptoms are protracted weight loss occurs as well. If the diagnosis is not made, the condition deteriorates, patients becoming drowsy; if they remained untreated, they would become comatose and eventually die.

Dehydration is the most obvious clinical feature of patients with ketoacidosis. They are also drowsy, but rarely unconscious although those with the most severe disorder may indeed be very gravely ill and unconscious too. The tongue looks like leather and the skin is inelastic as a result of dehydration. Overbreathing due to acidosis is usual, but patients are not normally breathless and the deep 'sighing' respiration (known as Kussmaul respiration after the man who first described it) is not always obvious. The breath smells of acetone although this is not always a valuable sign since many observers are unable to detect its scent. Most severe cases are hypothermic and features of circulatory collapse may be present, namely tachycardia, hypotension and peripheral vasoconstriction. Abdominal signs may include a gastric splash due to stasis, and bowel sounds are commonly reduced or even absent. Very rarely severe dehydration causes changes in the lens due to wrinkling of the capsule or streaks and clefts in the lens substance which disappear rapidly on rehydration.

When intercurrent illness has precipitated the episode of ketoacidosis there may be signs of other disorders. It is important to detect the presence of urinary tract infection, chest infection, infection of the feet and less commonly otitis media or meningitis. Myocardial infarction may have precipitated the event and the mortality is then about 50%.

Diagnosis

The diagnosis should be made clinically and treatment, at least with intravenous fluids, started immediately. The following tests are needed to confirm the diagnosis and establish the baseline from which to assess the effectiveness of treatment:

Blood glucose: Blood glucose concentrations in ketoacidosis span a very wide range but themselves give relatively little indication of the severity of the illness. They usually exceed 15 mmol/l (though lower levels are recorded) and are rarely above 80 mmol/l.

Blood acid base status: pH ranges from normal (in aketotic cases) to about 6.8. The bicarbonate value is depressed and ranges between 2 and 15 mmol/l.

Electrolytes: The initial serum potassium concentration is either normal or sometimes raised. This measurement is vital and lifesaving treatment is needed to maintain potassium values in the normal range. The sodium concentration is normal or reduced, the urea and creatinine concentrations often being raised as a result of dehydration.

Plasma ketones: These are easily detectable using ketostix on a plasma sample tested at the bedside. In patients with ketoacidosis the results of positive ketostix testing should be 2+ or 3+. The plasma ketostix text is useful if acidosis is thought to be due to another cause, such as lactic acidosis. The actual blood ketone levels (normally less than 0.2 mmol/l) may rise by 50-fold or more and are in the range 5–15 mmol/l in cases of ketoacidosis.

Blood count: There is often a leucocytosis which may be as high as 15–20 × 10^9/l even in the absence of infection.

Plasma osmolality: This is usually determined by the formula 2× [plasma sodium] + [urea] + [glucose] although it is preferably measured directly. It is always raised in ketoacidosis and 'aketotic hyperosmolar coma', the normal range being approximately 275–295 mOsmol/kg.

Urine: This should always show both heavy glycosuria and ketonuria.

Treatment

Diabetic ketoacidosis is a medical emergency with a significant mortality. Attention to these patients and treatment should never be delayed. The chief aspects of treatment can be summarized as follows: (1) intravenous fluids; (2) insertion of a nasogastric tube; (3) intravenous insulin; (4) correction of potassium depletion; (5) treatment of the underlying condition.

INTRAVENOUS FLUIDS

Fluid replacement is necessary and urgent in the treatment of these patients who are seriously dehydrated. Indeed the dehydration is usually so obvious that an intravenous drip should be set up immediately without waiting for biochemical results to be returned from the laboratory. The infusion rate needs to be rapid initially; if it is not, dehydration may persist and is aggravated by the passage of very large volumes of urine which result from the severe osmotic diuresis.

Normal saline (0.9%, 150 mmol/1) is given unless there is hyper-natraemia (serum sodium above 150 mmol/1) when half-normal saline (0.45%, 75 mmol/l) is used. The infusion rate generally recommended for a normal-weight adult is shown in Table 11.2. This may need to be modified especially in those with cardiac problems and then it is wise to monitor the intravenous therapy with a central venous line; if there is doubt about the cardiorespiratory state, a Swan–Ganz catheter is inserted.

Table 11.2 Fluid administration in diabetic ketoacidosis

Normal saline (150 mmol/l)	
1 litre in first half hour	0.5 h
1 litre over next hour	0.5–1.5 h
1 litre over next hour	1.5–2.5 h
1 litre over next 2 hours	2.5–4.5 h
1 litre over next 3 hours	4.5–7.5 h
1 litre over next 4 hours	7.5–11.5 h
Total 6 litres over	11.5 hours

1 These figures are for an average case in an average size (70 kg) person.
2 Fluid should be changed to dextrose 10% when blood glucose falls below 10 mmol/l.

In cases of severe hypotension plasma expanders may be needed, after obvious causes such as myocardial infarction have been excluded.

The fluid should be changed to dextrose 10% once the blood glucose concentration has fallen below 10 mmol/l. The rate of infusion is determined by individual need but at this stage should probably be about 1 litre every 8 hours.

Bicarbonate infusion: sodium bicarbonate infusion is not normally required and there is no good evidence for its efficacy. If, however, the blood pH is less than 7.0 or the patient is shocked then aliquots of sodium bicabonate (200 ml of 2.74% containing 65 mmol) may be given over 30–60 minutes. This can be repeated if there is no response within 1 hour and if the patient's condition remains serious. Administration of sodium bicarbonate accelerates hypokalaemia and, depending on the serum potassium concentration (see below), it is usual to add 15 mmol of potassium chloride to each 200 ml of sodium bicarbonate infused. High concentrations of sodium bicarbonate, such as the 8.4% used at cardiac arrest procedures, should *never* be given and are extremely dangerous.

INSERTION OF A NASOGASTRIC TUBE

This should always be performed if the patient is not fully conscious. The procedure is lifesaving and a small number of deaths still occur as a result of inhalation of gastric contents. Even those patients who are conscious should not be allowed to take any fluids by mouth since vomiting is almost inevitable. If patients complain bitterly of thirst, ice cubes may be given.

INSULIN TREATMENT

Soluble insulin is administered intravenously by constant infusion. It is normally given after diluting the soluble insulin at a concentration of 1.0 U/ml in normal saline and infused by a pump at 6 units per hour (0.1 U/kg/hour for children) until the blood glucose concentration is less than 10 mmol/l. Blood glucose should fall at a rate of about 5 mmol/l/hour (Fig. 11.2). Then the dose is reduced to 3 U/hour. If the blood glucose fails to fall it is important first to check that the infusion system is intact and working and that there are no leaking joints. If true insulin resistance is present the insulin infusion rate should be doubled (to 12 U/h) or subsequently quadrupled if necessary. The insulin infusion is continued until the patient is well enough to eat. Pre-prandial subcutaneous insulin is then given and intravenous insulin discontinued after the meal; it is usual to effect this change in the morning before breakfast and not at night when things tend to go wrong (see p. 108). Intravenous insulin has a very short half-life of only a

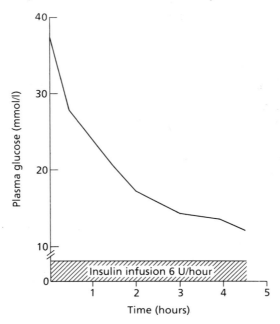

Fig. 11.2 The blood glucose response to i.v. insulin infusion, 6 U/hour in a case of ketoacidosis. The fall is steady at approx. 5 mmol/l/hour.

few minutes and should not be stopped before subcutaneous insulin has been given.

If the pump fails, if none is available or experience is lacking it is satisfactory to deliver the insulin intramuscularly. It is then usual to give soluble insulin 20 units as a loading dose and then 6 U/hour intramuscularly until the blood glucose is less than 10 mmol/l when it should be continued at 2-hourly intervals.

POTASSIUM ADMINISTRATION

Potassium chloride administration should usually start at about the second hour, and not before the serum potassium concentration is known unless there is certain ECG evidence of hypokalaemia. It should be withheld in the exceptional cases of oliguria or anuria or if the serum potassium value remains over 5 mmol/l. After the second hour, or earlier if the initial serum potassium value is normal or less than 4 mmol/l, potassium chloride should be added to each litre of saline according to the scale shown in Table 11.3. The exact amount should be determined by serum potassium measurements every 2 hours at first, then every 4 hours aiming to maintain the serum potassium between 4 and 5 mmol/l. Higher infusion rates of potassium are occasionally needed. An electrocardiographic monitor should always be set up and will show inversion of T-waves and/or development of U-waves if hypokalaemia occurs, or peaking in hyperkalaemia, but there is no substitute for serial potassium measurements.

Table 11.3 Approximate guide to potassium administration in diabetic ketoacidosis

Serum potassium (mmol/l)	Below 3.5	3.5–4.0	4.0–5.0	Above 5.0
Administration rate	40 mmol/l	30 mmol/l	20 mmol/l	Nil

1 See text for details.
2 Larger amounts are sometimes needed.

TREATMENT OF THE UNDERLYING CONDITION

Underlying disease should be sought; chest and urinary tract infections are the commonest. Blood and urine cultures, with a chest X-ray and ECG should be undertaken. Antibiotics are not given routinely unless there is reasonable evidence for the presence of infection, not simply a mild leucocytosis. Abdominal pain should always be taken seriously; the possibility of a genuine surgical acute abdomen needs to be considered. Although patients with ketoacidosis may experience some pain and tenderness, these features are rarely sufficient to cause confusion after careful examination.

Hyperosmolar aketotic diabetic coma

Insulin depletion is the cause of this condition just as it is for diabetic ketoacidosis, but probably because there is a small amount of residual insulin, ketogenesis is suppressed. It occurs most commonly in older patients and West Indians. Many cases develop in previously undiagnosed subjects. The blood glucose is sometimes very high, commonly over 60 mmol/l. Presentation is similar to that for ketoacidosis with profound dehydration as the most striking clinical feature. Patients are not normally comatose (the name is misleading) unless convulsions, rare but well recognized, have occurred; they can however present with stroke. Hyperketonaemia is slight, although ketonuria can occur; patients are not acidotic and do not, therefore, overbreathe. It is easy for the inexperienced to overlook the diagnosis and many patients are only detected after routine biochemistry results are returned from the laboratory. Treatment is the same as for ketoacidosis although if hypernatraemia exists (serum sodium greater than 150 mmol/l) it is usual to use half-normal saline (0.45%, 75 mmol/l) in the intravenous infusion. A lower rate of insulin infusion (3 U/hour) is often sufficient. Osmolality should be measured and may be extremely raised.

There is some additional hazard in these patients, from deep vein thrombosis and if the patients are very sick, low-dose subcutaneous heparin administration should be considered. After recovery many, but not all, of the patients prove to be non-insulin dependent; withdrawal of insulin must be undertaken very carefully since some patients relapse either immediately or after only a few weeks. Ketoacidosis and 'aketotic coma' can alternate in the same patient.

Lactic acidosis

Patients who develop lactic acidosis are usually profoundly ill from some other disorder causing shock and collapse. Metformin can cause lactic acidosis especially in patients with renal impairment and sometimes in those with liver disease or a high alcohol intake. The diagnosis should be considered whenever patients are profoundly sick and ketoacidosis can be confirmed or excluded by bedside assessment of plasma ketones using ketostix (see p. 100). Patients with lactic acidosis are very insulin-resistant and need very high rates of insulin infusion together with large amounts of sodium bicarbonate; the mortality is high.

Complications during treatment

While most patients given adequate treatment recover uneventfully, some serious if rare complications can occur.

Oliguria and anuria

Decline of renal function is relatively uncommon in patients with keto-acidosis, probably because of the powerful osmotic drive from hyper-glycaemia, so that even those who are severely dehydrated and hypotensive rarely become oliguric. If they do it is sometimes due to intercurrent renal disease, such as glomorulonephritis. Patients already affected by diabetic nephropathy also run into problems from rapid acceleration of their existing renal impairment. Rather more rarely patients with otherwise uncomplicated but exceptionally severe ketoacidosis, may develop tubular necrosis and renal failure requiring treatment in the usual ways, sometimes by dialysis, until recovery occurs.

Cerebral oedema

Some increase in intracranial pressure is probably not uncommon during the treatment of diabetic ketoacidosis. Occasionally this becomes very severe and florid cerebral oedema develops; the patient whose course during the first few hours appears uneventful gradually becomes stuporose as cerebral oedema develops. It is very important to exclude other causes for rising intracranial pressure since this complication is really very uncommon. It has been suggested that excessively rapid correction of the severe metabolic changes of ketoacidosis may accelerate cerebral oedema, but the true mechanism is obscure. It can be treated with mannitol and steroids but a few fatal cases have been reported.

Pulmonary oedema/adult respiratory distress syndrome (ARDS)

This occurs infrequently, usually when patients are over-hydrated, especially in the presence of existing cardiac disease. Caution should always be exercised during fluid administration in such patients and it is best always to monitor them with central venous pressure measurements, and ideally a Swan–Ganz catheter. Occasionally younger people inexplicably develop pulmonary oedema which may even require ventilation.

Disseminated intravascular coagulation

This is a rare but well-described hazard of ketoacidosis which may of course also be due to some other underlying disorder, including septicaemia. It presents in the usual way, and is normally first detected by the development of thrombocytopaenia followed by bruising and haematuria as well. The detection of fibrin degradation products in the urine establishes the diagnosis and administration of fresh frozen plasma is applied.

Thrombocytopaenia

An unexplained thrombocytopaenia sometimes develops independently of disseminated intravascular coagulation. It is due to phosphate depletion which is well known to occur as a result of diabetic ketoacidosis but rarely causes any problems. If thrombocytopaenia does occur and there is no other cause for it, it is reversed by phosphate infusion.

Prevention of diabetic ketoacidosis

Proper patient education is vital for the prevention of ketoacidosis. The most simple rule, namely that insulin should neither be reduced nor stopped during intercurrent illness, is still frequently disregarded. The management of diabetes during any illness is often difficult and needs to be well understood. It is discussed in detail on p. 86.

Management of diabetes during and after surgical operations and other emergencies

The chief principle of diabetic managment through any crisis in which patients cannot eat or drink for any reason is to continue insulin administration. It is best given by constant infusion either from the intravenous drip bag or by infusion pump. Insulin infusion can be continued more or less indefinitely by either of these methods and should continue until the patient is able to take food or fluids by mouth when subcutaneous insulin can be restarted.

These situations are frequently badly and dangerously managed. They require close cooperation between surgeon, anaesthetist and diabetic physician to prevent the occurrence of ketoacidosis or hypoglycaemia in the peri-operative period.

Some practical rules are:

1 For elective surgery diabetic patients should be placed first on a list wherever practical so that surgery takes place at a specific time.

2 Theatre staff, anaesthetists and ward nursing staff must always be informed that a patient is diabetic.

3 Details of their normal diabetic regimen must be written on the anaesthetic record.

4 There must be clear agreement as to which clinician is responsible for diabetic management at all stages.

5 High unacceptable blood glucose readings requiring immediate medical attention should be recorded in the notes.

6 The traditional sliding scale for insulin administration is obsolete.

Insulin-treated patients

One of the following procedures should be followed for all patients taking insulin, and for those whose NIDD has been poorly controlled (see below). The insulin pump technique is more suitable for the most complex procedures and allows for refinements of control independently of the intravenous drip regimen. Otherwise, resources or personal preference should determine the technique to be used.

GLUCOSE DRIP AND VARIABLE RATE INSULIN INFUSION (INSULIN PUMP)

1 Give usual subcutaneous insulin on evening before operation, but not on the morning of operation.

2 About 0800 h on day of operation, commence infusion of 10% glucose with added potassium chloride (20 mmol/l) and run at steady rate of 100 ml/hour. Start recording hourly blood glucose levels using 'stix' with a meter (not visual readings), having checked a laboratory blood glucose at the beginning.

3 Make up a solution of short-acting insulin (Actrapid, Velosulin, Humulins) at concentration of 1U/ml and infuse by syringe pump piggy-backed into the glucose infusion. The infusion rate shown on Scale 1 should

Table 11.4 Glucose drip and vaviable rate insulin infusion scales

	Insulin infusion rate (U/hour)		
Blood glucose	Scale 1	Scale 2	Scale 3
Below 4 mmol/l	0.5	1	2
4–10 mmol/1	2	4	8
Above 10 mmol/l	4	8	16
Above 17 mmol/l		Review individually	

normally be used, but may need to be increased to Scales 2 or 3 if the patient is resistant (e.g. severely ill patients, those previously on very high daily doses of insulin and those on steroids or sympathomimetics) (see Table 11.4).

Never stop insulin altogether (unless the patient is actually hypo-glycaemic) since intravenous insulin lasts for only a few minutes and hyperglycaemia is inevitable.

Urine tests including ketones should also be performed as a double check as should laboratory glucoses for values below 4 or above 17 mmol/l.

4 Blood glucose is measured preoperatively, then 2 hourly until stable, then 6-hourly.

Scale 1 is satisfactory for most cases; very severely-ill patients, those who are shocked and those on steroids or salbutamol infusions may need higher-dose infusions, such as regimens 2 or 3 and occasionally even more.

GLUCOSE–INSULIN INFUSION REGIMEN

This is preferable when no reliable pump is available or when staff are not practised in use of the pump.

1 Give the usual subcutaneous insulin on evening before operation, but not on the morning of operation.

2 Start recording hourly 'stix' using a meter (not visual readings), checking the first with a laboratory blood glucose.

3 Commence an infusion of 10% dextrose containing 16 U of short-acting insulin and 20 mmol/1 of potassium chloride. Run at 100 ml/hour.

If blood glucose remains between 4 and 10 mmol/l continue, otherwise make up new bags as shown in Table 11.5.

If 32 U/l is still insufficient to keep blood glucose below 17 mmol/l, review individually and increase insulin still further. A pump is better in insulin-resistant cases.

4 Urine tests including ketones should also be performed as a double check as should laboratory blood glucose levels for values below 4 or above 20 mmol/l.

Blood glucose is measured 2-hourly until stable, then 6 hourly. Urine tests should also be performed as a safeguard against erroneous ward blood glucose readings.

Table 11.5 Glucose–insulin infusion regimen

Blood glucose (mmol/l)	Insulin dose (U/l)
Less than 4	8
4–10	16
Above 10	32

AFTER RECOVERY

Once the patient starts to eat, soluble insulin should be given subcutaneously, usually three times daily. It is best to start this regimen in the morning before breakfast so that progress can be assessed while all normal staff are on duty. The intravenous insulin infusion should not be stopped until the subcutaneous insulin has been given otherwise the development of hyperglycaemia can be very rapid. If the previous dose of insulin is known it should be given in approximately three equal parts, although a larger total amount may be needed if the patient is still unwell or taking drugs such as steroids which cause insulin resistance. If the patient has not previously taken insulin it is reasonable to start soluble insulin at approximately 10 units tds. A sliding scale should never be used, but if blood glucose concentrations remain high (more than 15–17 mmol/l) the noon dose can be increased and if they are still high in the evening an additional dose can be given at bedtime. This regimen needs to be adjusted daily until blood glucose levels appear reasonable after which the definitive regimen can be commenced. This phase of diabetes treatment is often very badly handled by inexperienced, unsupervised junior staff who will always need help and advice from the diabetic team as to the details of management.

Non-insulin-dependent diabetics

Management of diabetics treated with diet or oral hypoglycaemic agents is more straightforward, so long as the diabetes is well controlled.

If the patient has well-controlled diabetes (random blood glucoses <12 mmol/l):

1 Omit oral hypoglycaemic on day of operation — care is needed with chlorpropamide and glibenclamide as these have a long half-life and the previous day's dose may still be effective.

2 Check laboratory blood glucose before and shortly after surgery with hourly meter readings in between. If below 4 mmol/l then commence glucose infusion (100 ml/hour of 10% dextrose); if above 10–12 mmol/l then commence insulin infusion or pump regimen (see above).

3 After surgery check blood glucose 1–2-hourly; restart oral hypoglycaemics before next normal meal, or insulin if control is unsatisfactory.

If the diabetes is poorly controlled (random blood glucoses > 12 mmol/l) the patient should be started on insulin before the operation, using one of the regimens described above.

Hypoglycaemia

Hypoglycaemia is a much commoner emergency than ketoacidosis and occurs at all grades of severity from the mild warning symptoms recognized by a patient and treated with immediate glucose and food to the deeply unconscious or physically aggressive casualty patient.

While the level at which patients feel unwell is variable it is rare for it to be a clinical problem above 2.5 mmol/l. The old practice of giving all new patients on insulin a deliberate 'hypo' is fortunately now past history. Hypoglycaemia can occur quite rapidly and remains much feared. It is necessary to reiterate that 'not waking up' and brain damage are incredibly rare in insulin-treated patients — counter-regulatory hormone responses and the relatively short life of most insulins tend to limit the duration of hypoglycaemia. The greatest danger is from accidents while driving a car.

Symptoms and signs

Most insulin-treated diabetics will experience early warning symptoms of hypoglycaemia moderately frequently and will take glucose appropriately. These are listed in Table 11.6 and tend to be specific for an individual; however, in later life awareness may be lost. This is also one of the effects of beta-blockers, which is a serious, though rare, practical problem. Friends, work colleagues and relatives are often more aware than the patient that he has become slow, vacant or withdrawn; he or she must learn to accept the prompting to eat! Loss of warning of hypoglycaemia is not always permanent and is not due to autonomic neuropathy.

A hypoglycaemic patient is typically pale, and may appear stupid or slow-witted. They may be aggressive and appear intoxicated. There are often tell-tale beads of perspiration on the brow, or the patient may be drenched from sweating. Night sweats from hypoglycaemia are described by some, and waking with headaches is another feature after nocturnal episodes. Deep coma can occur, during which the patient may be either limp or violent. Convulsions are not rare, especially in children, and laceration of the tongue or incontinence may then be observed. Hemiplegia is a rare feature which rapidly recovers when glucose is given.

Table 11.6 Symptoms and signs of hypoglycaemia

Early warning	Shaking, trembling
	Sweating
	Pins and needles in tongue and lips
	Palpitation
	Hunger
	Headache (especially early morning)
Neuroglycopenia	
Mild	Double vision
	Difficulty in concentration
	Slurring of speech
	Withdrawal/silence
Moderate	Confusion
	Change in behaviour
	Truculence
	Misbehaviour in children
Late	Restlessness with sweating
	Epileptic fits, especially children
	Hemiplegia in elderly (rare and reversible)

Hypoglycaemia can occur at any time, but most frequently during the late morning before the mid-day meal and during the night. At night the patient either wakes of his or her own accord, or his or her spouse may wake in response to restlessness or sweating. Sugar should be available at the bedside. Patients do not always recollect events during hypoglycaemia and can sometimes perform acts of which they are quite unaware; some have even driven their cars for several miles without any recollection! Minor offences can sometimes be committed unwittingly during hypoglycaemia (Chapter 22, p. 230).

Causes of hypoglycaemia

Precipitating causes of hypoglycaemia are too much insulin, delayed meals, insufficient carbohydrate (particularly between-meal snacks) and increased exercise. The severity of hypoglycaemia can be gauged, not only by blood glucose measurement, but by the extent of assistance needed. Thus the simplest episodes are dealt with by the patient himself, more severe episodes need the assistance of relatives or friends while the worst attacks require professional attention with or without intravenous glucose. If glucose fails, the patient should be taken to the nearest available doctor or casualty department.

Treatment

1 Confirmation of hypoglycaemia. Confirmation of the diagnosis is essential, especially if the episode is severe, but should not delay treatment. While glucose sticks are helpful they should not be relied upon in this situation and a laboratory blood glucose should be obtained.

2 Immediate correction of hypoglycaemia. If the patient is conscious then oral glucose as a drink, tablet or gel can be used (Table 11.7). If he is not intravenous glucose should be given, commonly 20–50 ml of 50% glucose. This hypertonic solution is very irritant and must be given carefully into a vein. The response is usually immediate but, if not, a further dose should be

Table 11.7 Suitable treatment for hypoglycaemia

Lucozade	60 ml (2 fl oz)
Ribena	15 ml (0.5 fl oz)
Coca-cola (not Diet)	80 ml (3 fl oz)
Sugar	2 teaspoons
Sugar lumps	3 small
Dextrosol	3 tablets

Each item contains 10 g of carbohydrate.

given after 5 min followed by an infusion of 10% glucose. If recovery does not occur rapidly, another cause for the coma must be sought. If hypoglycaemia has been profound, cerebral oedema can occur and may require treatment with dexamethasone or mannitol.

If intravenous access cannot be obtained then intramuscular glucagon should be given (1 mg from a kit); this requires adequate liver glycogen stores and should never be used repeatedly. It is however a valuable standby for those patients with recurrent hypoglycaemia for whom a trained family member can give the injection. Large stocks should not be given.

3 Prevention of recurrent hypoglycaemia. Once full consciousness is restored and a history can be taken, the patient should be fed with longer-acting carbohydrate to prevent recurrence.

When oral hypoglycaemics are the cause the patient should be admitted as these agents, especially chlorpropamide and glibenclamide, can continue to produce hypoglycaemia over 24–48 hours.

4 Long-term prevention of hypoglycaemia. Any hypoglycaemic attack is, to some extent, a failure of doctor, patient or regimen. It should provoke a brief enquiry to establish the cause and to see if it is likely to recur (p. 111). Where nocturnal hypoglycaemia is a problem, a few blood tests at the usual time (using an alarm clock) can be useful.

The opportunity for necessary education should be taken, in particular to ensure that any patient taking insulin always carries some form of glucose or sugar with them together with a diabetic identification card.

Further reading

Refer to major textbooks and see general reading list on p. 240.

Section 3
Diabetic Complications

12: An Overview of Complications

After the discovery of insulin which both saved life and improved its quality, it rapidly became clear that diabetes was not just an acute metabolic threat to life but also caused chronic complications, some of which could themselves lead to premature death or disability. It was thus only in the late 1920s and 1930s that the scale of these became obvious and detailed descriptions of the syndromes were made. There are both complications specific to diabetes such as retinopathy and other non-specific problems which occur with increased frequency in diabetes, notably coronary heart disease; these are listed in Table 12.1. The epidemiology of the individual complications is discussed in the separate chapters.

Pathogenesis of diabetic complications

The major organs most affected by diabetes are the eye, the kidney and peripheral nerves, but no single explanation of the pathogenesis of these complications is possible as the individual organs are indeed affected to a very different extent; at times disease in one tissue is advanced while another is spared altogether.

The major theories regarding the development of complications are based on metabolic and vascular changes; these are not mutually exclusive since metabolic changes can give rise to altered vascularity. They have proved difficult to investigate and substantiate and animal models are imperfect.

Many attempts have been made to establish clear genetic markers of susceptibility to particular complications. These include HLA status, complement factors and chromosomal markers. As yet no definite markers of any clinical relevance have been identified.

The ultrastructural change of basement membrane thickening is the hallmark of long-standing diabetes; it is seen in many tissues including the kidney, retina and nerve, and is also observed in skin, muscle and adipose tissue. It is closely related to the duration of diabetes, but its relationship to functional abnormalities is less clear.

Biochemical abnormalities may also be important in the pathogenesis of complications. In particular, recent observations regarding glycation

115

Table 12.1 The major complications of diabetes

Specific complications	*Increased frequency of other diseases*
Renal disease	Cardiac problems
Diabetic nephropathy	Coronary heart disease
Eye disease	Eyes
Background retinopathy	Cataracts
Proliferative retinopathy	Nerves
Neuropathy	Carpal tunnel syndrome
Peripheral neuropathies	
Autonomic neuropathy	
Cranial nerve palsies	
Peripheral mononeuropathies	
Skin complications	
Necrobiosis lipoidica	
Joint complications	
Diabetic cheiroarthropathy	

(glycosylation) of proteins and the sorbitol–inositol pathway, with an intracellular accumulation of sorbitol, have aroused considerable interest.

Glycation of proteins

Glucose binds to many proteins, mainly linking to lysine residues, and the extent of the reaction depends upon the prevailing glucose concentration. This initial reaction then undergoes a rearrangement to form a more permanent product. Glycated haemoglobin (HbA1$_c$ or HbA 1 — p. 47) is used to provide a measure of mean glycaemic control. The idea that glycated material behaves differently and may interfere with its normal function or breakdown is of particular interest. Enzyme activity may be altered in this way and physical properties (e.g. cell rigidity) actually changed, for example in the Schwann cell basal lamina in peripheral nerves.

More detailed consideration of the pathogenesis of individual complications will be found in the individual chapters.

Diabetic control and complications

Diabetic control, expressed by any glycaemic index such as mean blood glucose or HBA1, is strongly related to the development of retinopathy, nephropathy and peripheral neuropathy. This observation does not however prove that hyperglycaemia is their direct cause, nor that improvement of control will automatically diminish them.

Very large scale randomized studies of optimal compared with conventional glycaemic control are now in progress in the USA (the Diabetic

Control and Complications Trial) but numerous intensive studies on established diabetics have suggested the following:

1 Long-term improved control reduces the progression of established peripheral neuropathy, early to moderate retinopathy and very early nephropathy but has much less effect, if any, on more advanced stages of these problems. The beneficial effects are usually apparent only after a year or two and show slowing of the rate of damage and rarely its reversal.

2 Acute improvements of previously poor control may worsen pre-existing retinopathy. The appearance of cotton wool spots is the commonest phenomenon and is usually seen in the weeks or months after the tightening of control; these changes disappear within about 2 years. Acute development of proliferative retinopathy and vitreous haemorrhage can occur but is fortunately rare.

3 Glycaemic control has not been shown to affect the development of macrovascular disease.

One further important point is that those who do not attend regularly for medical attention have a very high rate of complications; whether this reflects just poor control or other risk factors is not clear.

Duration of diabetes and complications

The chronic complications of IDD namely retinopathy, nephropathy and autonomic and peripheral neuropathy are rarely seen before 5–7 years duration of diabetes and occur most commonly after 10–20 years. However, NIDD patients not infrequently present with retinopathy, neuropathy or foot ulceration. This is because NIDD has almost certainly been present for several years before presentation. The strategy for screening for complications in patients with NIDD must be considered from the time of presentation when these patients are already at risk. Complications continue to increase as duration of diabetes lengthens, but after 30 years their annual incidence appears to decrease. Some diabetics are free from complications after 40, 50 or even 60 years.

Association of complications

IDD

In IDD, almost all patients (over 95%) with nephropathy have background or proliferative retinopathy. However, patients with retinopathy or neuropathy do not invariably have nephropathy. Both peripheral and autonomic neuropathy are much commoner in those with nephropathy and retinopathy than in those without. Neuropathies however sometimes develop in those with no other complications. The common relationships are shown in Fig. 12.1.

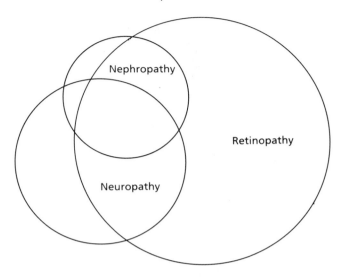

Fig. 12.1 Venn diagram of microvascular complications in IDD.

Macrovascular disease (especially coronary artery disease) in those with IDD is much commoner among patients with nephropathy (detailed discussion in Chapter 13). Persistent proteinuria is the best single marker of the risk for mortality. The risk of macrovascular disease in diabetics free from proteinuria, though higher than normal, is very much less than that found in the patients with nephropathy (Fig. 16.1).

NON-INSULIN-DEPENDENT DIABETES

In NIDD, the patterns are less clear. The relationship between proteinuria and macrovascular disease is strong; retinopathy and neuropathy are also commoner in this group although the association is less striking than in IDD. Isolated retinopathy or neuropathy also occur. The best marker for mortality usually from coronary artery disease is proteinuria (see Chapter 16).

Early detection of diabetic complications

A major difficulty in the early detection of diabetic complications is that most are symptomless until an advanced stage. The earliest changes are only detectable on careful clinical or laboratory examination and changes have to be advanced before the patient is aware that anything is wrong (Table 12.2). Similarly, patients may be unaware of a sensory peripheral

Table 12.2 Signs, symptoms and early detection methods of complications

Complication	Earliest symptom	Earliest sign	Early detection
Retinopathy	Poor vision	Retinal changes	Regular screening Photography
Nephropathy	Nausea, anorexia, itching	Signs of ESRF	'Microalbuminuria'
Neuropathy	Parasthesiae	Vibration or temperature abnormalities	Biothesiometer

neuropathy until the development of a foot lesion, and major changes in autonomic function tests may long precede any complaints from the patient.

The clinical presentation of macrovascular disease obviously assumes importance with the development of angina or myocardial infarction, claudication or gangrene, and transient ischaemic attacks or strokes. Advanced arterial disease must however have been present for many years before clinical presentation. The emphasis now has changed from treatment of established complications to screening, early detection and aggressive early therapy.

Subsequent chapters will deal with each complication in turn, and will include mention of modern strategies for the early detection of these complications.

Further reading

Keen H. & Jarrett J. (1982). *Diabetes and its Complications*, 2nd edn. Edward Arnold, London
Panzram G. (1987). Mortality and survival in Type 2 (non-insulin-dependent) diabetes. *Diabetologia*, **30**, 123–131

13: Diabetic Renal Disease (Nephropathy)

Diabetic nephropathy is a specific renal disease affecting a significant proportion of all diabetics and is responsible for 15–25% of all end-stage renal failure in patients in Western countries. While IDD is responsible for the majority of cases under 50 years of age, the problem is being increasingly recognized in older NIDD patients, especially those of Asian or Afro-Caribbean origin.

Diagnosis

The clinical diagnosis of diabetic nephropathy in IDD relies on the following features:

1 Detection of persistent proteinuria after more than 7–10 years of diabetes.

2 The presence of diabetic retinopathy of any severity.

3 The absence of evidence of other causes of renal disease, urinary tract infection or heart failure.

The diagnosis in NIDD is more difficult as proteinuria is common but does not necessarily imply progressive renal impairment; additionally proteinuria and nephropathy may occur in these patients at any time after diagnosis.

Persistent proteinuria is defined as positive Albustix (or other similar sticks) readings on at least three occasions over a period of 6 months and as the excretion of more than 500 mg of protein or 300 mg of albumin in 24 hours. A history of other renal disease militates against diabetic nephropathy as do haematuria, unequally sized, misshapen or very small kidneys and the absence of other diabetic complications.

Biopsy may be necessary in doubtful cases to exclude other causes of renal disease. Some diabetic changes (e.g. arteriolohyalinosis and glomerulosclerosis) are present in most subjects with over 10 years of diabetes; only increased glomerular mesangium and interstitial tissue, and the number of open glomerular capillaries correlate well with renal function (Fig. 13.1).

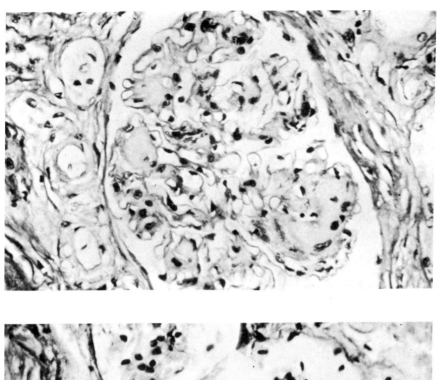

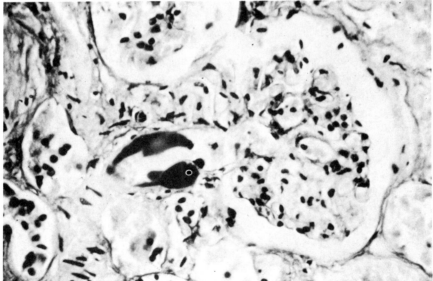

Fig. 13.1 Microscopic appearances of diabetic nephropathy showing glomerulosclerosis, mesangial thickening and closed glomerular capillaries.

Possible causes

There is a clear and strong association between poor control and the occurrence of nephropathy in both IDD and NIDD from both cross-sectional and prospective data, with a risk ratio from worst to best control of at least 5:1 and probably more. However it is still possible for a well-controlled patient to develop nephropathy and for another, always appallingly controlled, to escape it. Other factors must also operate however as a similar relationship exists between control and retinopathy; yet many patients develop retinopathy but not nephropathy.

No genetic markers for susceptibility had been identified until recently when an association between increased sodium–lithium countertransport and diabetic renal disease was demonstrated. One suggestion has been that pre-existing hypertension favours the development of nephropathy but this has not been substantiated.

Natural history of diabetic nephropathy

Insulin-dependent diabetes

There is an increasing incidence of nephropathy after 7–10 years of diabetes rising to a peak at 15–20 years, later falling considerably (Fig. 13.2); few patients develop it after 30 years of diabetes. In all 30–50% of patients develop nephropathy. There is an increased incidence in those diagnosed before age 20 and in males, as for other renal diseases. In recent years there appears to be a fall in the proportion of those developing nephropathy.

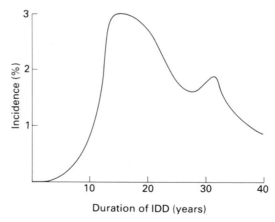

Fig. 13.2 The incidence of diabetic nephropathy with increasing duration of IDD. The second peak is not confirmed in all studies (from Andersen A.R. *et al.* (1983). *Diabetologia*, **25**, 496–501).

Much more is now known about the early stages of diabetic renal disease (Table 13.1) and the transition from normal kidneys to established renal disease. It must be emphasized that the process is completely asymptomatic until quite an advanced stage of renal failure, and detection is therefore only possible by regular urine examination; the usual dipsticks (e.g. albustix) only become positive at about 150 mg/1 of albumin and are very dependent on the observer.

EARLY DIABETES

In IDD there are several abnormalities of renal structure and function. The kidneys are large and, as a group, show higher glomerular filtration rates than normal — 'hyperfiltration'. This is partly, but not wholly, related to poor glycaemic control of the diabetes.

Protein excretion, in particular of albumin, is normal at this stage; excretion is now measured by sensitive assays which can detect down to 1 mg/l of albumin, less than the levels seen in non-diabetic people where the normal range extends up to about 25 mg/l or per 24 hours, though there is wide variability. Important decisions should never be made on a single result.

Blood pressure in these diabetic subjects is essentially normal, usually around 120/75 mmHg.

'INCIPIENT NEPHROPATHY' OR 'MICROALBUMINURIA'

These two terms are essentially synonymous, and describe the earliest stage of definite damage to the kidney though still with normal glomerular filtration rate (GFR). 'Microalbuminuria' refers to micro-amounts of albumin in the urine, not to a protein called 'microalbumin'! This stage only occurs after at least 5 years of IDD and refers to an albumin excretion of approximately 30–200 μg/min; exact levels vary depending on the urine collection used (24 hours, overnight timed etc).

Though GFR is normal, these patients have marginally raised blood pressures (about 135/85 mmHg) compared with those who are free from microalbuminuria. The real significance of microalbuminuria in IDD is that it usually predicts later development of clinical nephropathy and end-stage renal failure though it may not always do so.

PERSISTENT PROTEINURIA

Once persistent proteinuria is present, with loss of over 500 mg of protein or 200–300 mg/day of albumin, GFR falls progressively and relentlessly such

Table 13.1 The progression of diabetic nephropathy in IDD

Stage of disease	Glomerular filtration rate (GFR)	Albumin excretion	Blood pressure
No nephropathy	Normal to high (hyperfiltration)	Normal	Normal, e.g. 120/75 mmHg
'Microalbuminuria' or incipient nephropathy	Normal to high	Raised 30–200 μg/min	Slightly elevated, e.g. 135/85
Persistent proteinuria ⎫	Normal to low (declining)	High >300 μg/min (total protein >0.5 g/day)	High and rising, e.g. 145/95
Clinical nephropathy ⎬			
End-stage renal failure	<20 ml/min approx.	High, but often falls in late stage	High, e.g. 160/100

that end-stage renal failure is reached in an average of 7–10 years. Individuals however vary widely in the rate of decline. Blood pressure at this stage averages 145/95 mmHg and many patients have left ventricular hypertrophy on echocardiogram as well as slightly higher cholesterol levels. Some degree of retinopathy is almost invariable in these patients but the reverse is not true; it is quite possible to have advanced retinopathy, either background or proliferative, without any renal abnormality.

EARLY RENAL IMPAIRMENT

Persistent proteinuria continues, and tends to increase, as GFR falls progressively but true nephrotic syndrome is not common. Serum creatinine may increase from 200 μmol/l to end-stage renal failure in 6 months or may take 20 years. Other diabetic complications are very common in this group, especially peripheral and autonomic neuropathy and especially peripheral vascular disease. Clinical coronary heart disease, with angina and myocardial infarction, becomes common.

END-STAGE RENAL FAILURE

At this stage patients become symptomatic. This appears to happen in diabetes at a lower creatinine level than for non-diabetics. Management is described below.

Blood pressure at this stage is usually 160/100 mmHg or more, and extensive micro- and macrovascular complications are the rule. A significant proportion of patients are blind from proliferative retinopathy, and others have suffered myocardial infarction or amputations from the effects of peripheral vascular disease (see below).

Non-insulin-dependent diabetes

Proteinuria in NIDD is of less specificity than in IDD. It may be present at the time of diagnosis and patients with 'persistent' proteinuria do not necessarily proceed to develop abnormal renal function as measured by GFR or serum creatinine, even when the proteinuria increases. The associations of proteinuria with other complications, such as retinopathy, and with hypertension are much less marked than in patients with IDD and few die of chronic renal failure. However Asian and Afro-Caribbean patients with NIDD do have an increased risk of developing both proteinuria and renal failure and form as many as 50% of the NIDD patients reaching end-stage renal failure. The excess risk above the Caucasian population is difficult to quantify but is probably at least five-fold.

Proteinuria in NIDD, even microalbuminuria, is however associated with a higher overall mortality than in non-proteinuric subjects, mainly from cardiovascular disease.

Detection and investigation

It is obviously vital to detect diabetic nephropathy as early as possible to allow treatment before there is significant loss of renal function. The importance of regular checks of the urine for protein or albumin is obvious though the insensitivity of albustix must be recognized; routine screening for microalbuminuria on early morning or random samples should become normal practice.

Poorly controlled patients and those who are infrequent attenders are at high risk, while those with proliferative or severe background retinopathy and those with hypertension or increasing blood pressure should be checked especially carefully.

If albuminuria is detected, without other obvious cause, the following investigations are recommended:
1   Check on the history for other renal disease.
2   A mid-stream urine specimen for culture and microscopy.
3   Ultrasound examination of the kidneys.
4   Measurement of serum creatinine, and comparison with previous levels.
5   Blood pressure measurement, with ECG and chest X-ray if raised.
6   A 24-hour or timed overnight urine collection (single sample not adequate).
7   Careful fundal examination.

If increased albumin excretion or persistent proteinuria is confirmed then many patients will need further renal investigations such as anti-nuclear factor and complement levels, together with bladder assessment if indicated. Renal biopsy is usually only performed where there are discrepancies or doubt, or if the renal disease is of acute onset.

Factors influencing progression of nephropathy

Glycaemic control, dietary protein intake and blood pressure levels may be important in determining the rate of deterioriation; blood pressure appears to be the most important.

Glycaemic control

Microalbuminuria may be reduced by good glycaemic control but later in the disease it appears that even very good glycaemic control makes little or no difference to the rate of decline of GFR.

Anti-hypertensive therapy

There is strong, but not conclusive, evidence that anti-hypertensive therapy at the stage of persistent proteinuria or established nephropathy slows the progression of the renal disease and reduces albuminuria. In the longest study so far performed the rate of decline of GFR fell by over 80%. The early studies were performed with beta-blockers (usually metoprolol), diuretics (bendrofluazide/frusemide) and vasodilators (usually hydrallazine). More recently the converting enzyme inhibitors, captopril and enalapril, have been employed with frusemide; these have the advantages of being better tolerated in many patients, and the diuretic decreases the sodium and water retention which is so common in these patients. Blood pressure control to achieve these results has to be rigorous, a pressure well below 140/90 mmHg, but abrupt falls in blood pressure must be avoided as they can cause acute deterioration in renal function.

Protein restriction

Dietary protein restriction slows the progression of other renal diseases and may well do the same in diabetic nephropathy, though the benefit is smaller than for anti-hypertensive therapy. Restriction to 40–50 g/day is difficult to achieve, or for patients to tolerate for any length of time. Reduction to about 60 g/day is more practicable and dietary protein assessment is worthwhile to detect those with very high protein intakes which should be reduced.

Complications and mortality

Mortality

The marked increase in the rate of mortality among patients with IDD occurs predominantly amongst those who develop nephropathy (proteinuria), the main cause of death being myocardial infarction. IDD patients without proteinuria have a mortality rate of about twice that of a non-diabetic population while those with proteinuria have relative mortality rates of up to 100-fold. There are also considerable excesses in the frequency of retinopathy, blindness and neuropathy. Even amongst young patients with nephropathy, about 25% die from myocardial infarction before reaching end-stage renal failure while the majority of the older NIDD patients with nephropathy die from this cause rather than renal failure.

Complications

These do not differ from those described in Chapters 12–17, but a brief consideration here is worthwhile.

CARDIAC DISEASE IN DIABETIC NEPHROPATHY

Coronary arteriograms in patients reaching end-stage renal failure (ESRF) show that 25–40% have severe coronary disease, 20% are known to have had myocardial infarcts and over 50% have abnormal electrocardiograms.

CEREBROVASCULAR AND PERIPHERAL VASCULAR DISEASE

Up to 10% of patients in end-stage renal failure, mainly those with NIDD, have had disabling strokes and about 5% have had amputations. Arterial calcification is common and extensive and gangrene commonly affects toes and even fingers.

RETINOPATHY

Retinopathy precedes proteinuria in most patients, and indeed the absence of retinopathy should prompt reconsideration of the diagnosis. Over 75% of patients with advanced renal failure have proliferative retinopathy and 25–30% are blind. Retinopathy continues to progress even after successful dialysis or transplantation, with continuing neo-vascularization; frequent examination and energetic photocoagulation for new lesions are necessary.

NEUROPATHY

Diabetic neuropathy is present in most patients reaching advanced nephropathy, though the severity varies considerably from asymptomatic patients to those devastated by the problems of peripheral or autonomic neuropathy. The chief problems are the development of foot ulcers, sepsis and digital gangrene. Charcot neuroarthropathic joints and neuropathic oedema also occur. Foot problems are much more serious in the presence of peripheral vascular disease which must be actively treated.

Autonomic neuropathy is almost universally detectable in advanced nephropathy patients. Gustatory sweating is common, and sometimes remits after transplantation. Serious problems from postural hypotension and failure of bladder emptying are fortunately rare, but disabling when they occur.

Management of patients reaching end-stage renal failure

Only in the last decade have diabetic patients with end-stage renal failure been widely accepted onto transplantation and dialysis programmes in the

UK and it still appears that they are somewhat under-represented; other countries have far better records. About 60–70% of young insulin-dependent patients who develop nephropathy will die in end-stage renal failure if left untreated, with a male preponderance of 5 : 3. Among the NIDD group, Asian and Afro-Caribbean patients form a large proportion of the patients.

Once renal function is significantly impaired, ideal management is by joint care from both diabetic and renal physicians; early collaboration allows thorough investigation and treatment of the many facets of the disease and eventually ensures a smoother transition to renal support treatment.

Special attention is given to problems from hypertension and fluid retention which probably occur earlier than in other renal diseases. Retinopathy should be monitored closely, in particular arranging photo-coagulation when appropriate. The possibility of urinary tract infection should be checked and bladder emptying assessed by ultrasound. Biochemical analysis detects the development of hypo-albuminaemia and metabolic bone disease.

Progress is assessed by measuring serum creatinine levels — the inverse creatinine ratio (1/creatinine) is an approximation to the GFR and, in the untreated patient, shows a linear decline with time. An estimated GFR can be calculated using the formulae:

[88(145 — age in years)/(serum creatinine) — 3] for men
[75(145 — age in years)/(serum creatinine) — 3] for women

All diabetics developing renal failure should be considered for renal support treatment. Occasionally this is contraindicated because of over-whelming complications notably from cardiovascular or cerebrovascular disease, senility or carcinomatosis. Blindness alone is not a contraindication.

Over 80% of such patients are suitable for treatment. Many who appear initially to be poor prospects manage extremely well with good training and obtain a very satisfactory quality of life.

Indications for commencing treatment are the development of uraemic symptoms, notably malaise, nausea or anorexia, itching or fluid retention, or a serum creatinine > c. 450–550 μmol/l or a GFR < 20 ml/min.

Renal support treatments

Renal transplantation is the treatment of choice. With the present shortage of donor kidneys this can unfortunately rarely be achieved as the first treatment, and most diabetics start on continuous ambulatory peritoneal dialysis (CAPD); only a few start on haemodialysis. Starting treatment with dialysis permits a detailed assessment regarding suitability for trans-plantation.

Continuous ambulatory peritoneal dialysis

Continuous ambulatory peritoneal dialysis (CAPD) is relatively simple and can be used either to maintain health until transplantation is possible or as a definitive therapy. Two-year survival is now comparable to that for transplantation and is about 75% for both IDD and NIDD patients, and probably rather better than for haemodialysis.

One advantage in CAPD is the very simple technique of intraperitoneal insulin administration. Insulin is well absorbed from the peritoneum and during 6 hours about 50% of 15–20 units will disappear. Overall the total dose required is usually more than the subcutaneous dose; initially one-quarter of the daily dose is injected into each 6-hour bag, and adjustments made thereafter on the basis of home blood glucose measurements performed before each bag is changed. Glucose absorption and hyper-glycaemia are considerable when bags containing 3.86% glucose are used and more insulin is needed than in those with 1.36% glucose; rather less, perhaps half the amount of insulin, is needed in bags used overnight.

If peritonitis or other intercurrent illness develops, uncontrolled diabetes is best treated by intravenous insulin infusion.

Transplantation

The outcome for renal transplantation has progressively improved during the last decade. With cadaver transplants overall 2-year survival is about 90% for non-diabetics and about 75% for diabetics. Organ survival is comparable to patient survival, over 70% after 2 years. Diabetic complications, especially vascular disease, account for the poorer results for diabetics; mortality rates are much higher when there is severe ischaemic heart disease or heart failure. After transplantation myocardial infarction is responsible for 30–50% of deaths, significantly more than amongst non-diabetics. While the remainder of early deaths are mainly from infection, deaths beyond 2 years after transplantation are mostly from heart disease. 10 years after transplantation 20% have suffered myocardial infarction, 15% strokes and 30% amputations.

Management of diabetes and its complications

Intravenous insulin infusion is always used during surgery and when intercurrent infections develop; it is also needed in addition to subcutaneous insulin if rejection episodes require high-dose steroids. Routine treatment after recovery is best undertaken using a short-acting insulin preparation before each main meal (insulin pen devices are invaluable) and a longer-acting insulin at bed-time; this regimen is very flexible.

Diabetic complications continue to develop after successful transplantation, and joint care by renal and diabetic physicians is essential.

Conclusions

Since the last edition of this book there have been dramatic improvements to the outlook for patients with diabetic renal disease — transplantation or CAPD are now available for the great majority of patients with end-stage renal failure though they still have a high mortality rate and large chance of other complications.

Further reading

Brenner B.M. & Stein J.H. (eds) (1989). *The Kidney in Diabetes Mellitus*. Churchill Livingstone, New York

Drury P.L., Watkins P.J., Viberti G.C. & Walker J.D. (1989). Diabetic nephropathy. *British Medical Bulletin*, **45**, 127–147

Mogensen C.E. (ed) (1988). *The Kidney and Hypertension in Diabetes Mellitus*. Martinus Nijhoff Publishing, Boston

14: Diabetic Eye Disease

Blindness is one of most feared complications of diabetes. It is caused by a specific retinopathy, from excessive cataract formation occuring in diabetics or more rarely from rubeotic glaucoma. While retinopathy develops in most, though not all, diabetics of long duration, blindness occurs in up to 12% of IDD patients and 5% of NIDD patients after 30 years of diabetes. Because diabetes is very common, diabetic retinopathy is overall one of the four commonest causes of blindess in the community together with cataract, glaucoma and senile macular degeneration. Most blind diabetics are over 60 years of age.

Retinopathy

Retinopathy usually develops insidiously over many years. It is infrequently present before 7–10 years of diabetes in IDD patients although in NIDD it becomes increasingly common at diagnosis especially in older patients. After 20 years of diabetes, more than 80% of IDD patients have some degree of retinopathy and almost half of all patients with NIDD show changes after 15 years. In many cases this is a mild background retinopathy which changes little over many years. Rather unpredictably however, changes may develop which threaten vision either from macular disease or from vitreous haemorrhage in proliferative retinopathy. Maculopathy develops insidiously and is predominantly a disease of NIDD, while proliferative retinopathy occurs more frequently in people with IDD, half developing this form of disease after 15 years compared with only 20% of NIDD patients (Fig. 14.1).

It is not known why in some cases progression is very slow and in others terrifyingly fast. It is not simply the result of diabetic control. Paradoxically, in a very few instances, severe tightening of diabetic control after long periods of hyperglycaemia may cause rapid development of neo-vascularization with vitreous haemorrhages and blindness over a very short period of time. These unpleasant accelerated changes are sometimes described as 'bush-fire retinopathy'.

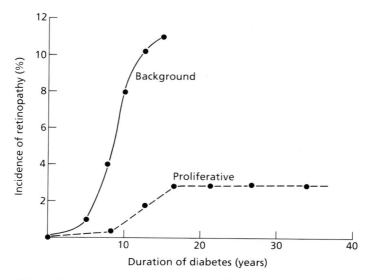

Fig. 14.1 The incidence of retinopathy in a cohort of IDD patients.

Pathophysiology

Capillary abnormalities are the earliest changes to occur in diabetes; small areas of capillary closure with associated retinal non-perfusion can be seen using fluorescein angiography with retinal photography (Fig. 14.2). The areas of non-perfusion increase in size until visible lesions appear. Subsequently arteriolar and arterial occlusion may develop and areas of non-perfusion increase still further.

The cause of these early abnormalities is not well understood. Endothelial cell proliferation and then degeneration occur; capillary closure is associated with disappearance of the endothelial cells. The underlying abnormalities are numerous. There may be an early increase of retinal blood-flow, there are numerous coagulation abnormalities and biochemical abnormalities with, for example, an accumulation of sorbitol (see p. 46) in the vessel wall.

Capillary closure and retinal ischaemia result in excessive leakage from diseased capillaries well seen using fluorescein angiography. When this is severe, maculopathy and macular oedema can occur. Ischaemic areas may be seen as cotton wool spots, and provide the stimulus to the growth of new vessels. The nature of the 'angiogenic' factor is still uncertain. Elevated blood levels of insulin-like growth factors (somatomedins) have been reported in some patients with rapidly advancing proliferative retinopathy. The theoretical basis for laser photocoagulation treatment in proliferative

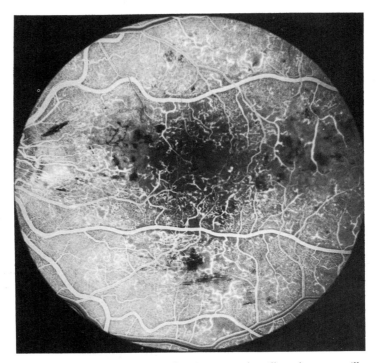

Fig. 14.2 Retinal fluorescein angiogram showing areas of capillary closure, capillary leakage and microaneurysms.

retinopathy is the destruction of ischaemic retina thereby reducing the release of the 'angiogenic' factor.

EARLY CHANGES

There are unconfirmed observations suggesting an early breakdown of the blood–retinal barrier with leakage of fluorescein into the vitreous. Increased retinal blood flow may also be an early feature of diabetes.

Background retinopathy

Microaneurysms (Plate 1) are the earliest recognizable abnormalities of diabetic retinopathy. They represent minute bulges or dilatations of retinal capillaries. They appear as tiny red dots; more of them are seen using the technique of fluorescein angiography. They are abnormally permeable but by themselves not harmful.

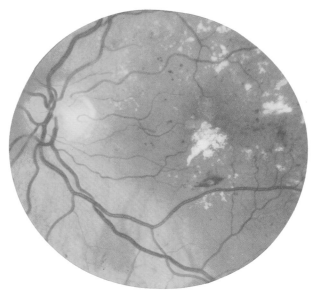

Plate 1 Extensive background retinopathy with multiple microaneurysms ('dots'), 'blot' haemorrhages and many hard exudates, especially in the ring surrounding the macula. This is especially common in NIDD and is often associated with macular oedema; it presents a major hazard to vision.

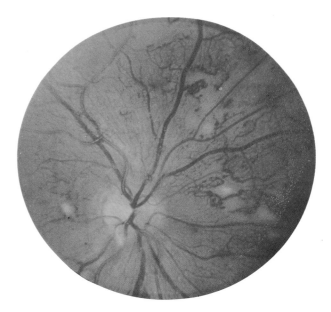

Plate 2 This illustrates extensive intraretinal microvascular abnormalities (IRMA) with some new vessel formation elsewhere (NVE) and cotton wool spots, best seen at 9 o'clock to the disc. There are also extensive microaneurysms and blot haemorrhages.

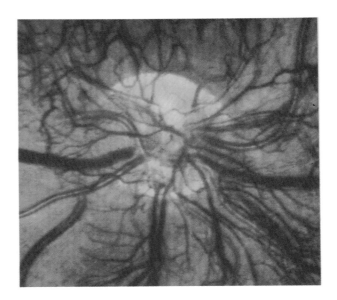

Plate 3 Extensive new vessels arising from the disc.

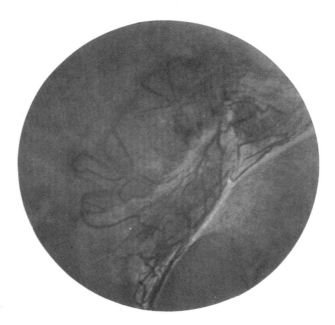

Plate 4 This shows extensive new vessel formation (retinitis proliferans) growing forward into the vitreous and subsequent fibrosis, the crescentic line, which has pulled the retina away.

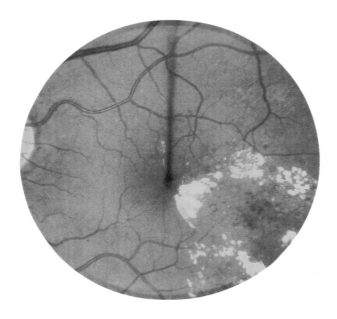

Plate 5

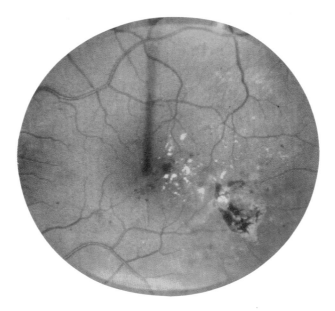

Plates 5 and 6 Successful treatment with photocoagulation — the appearances of active background retinopathy before (Plate 5) and after (Plate 6) photocoagulation. In the second picture pigmented scars in the areas of retinal ablation can be seen.

'Hard' exudates

These are yellow-white discrete patches of lipid which often occur in rings around leaking capillaries (Plate 1). They may coalesce to form extensive sheets of exudate. They cause blindness only when they develop on the macula.

Haemorrhages

These appear as small (dot) and large (blot) red spots on the retina (Plate 1). They harm vision when they appear on the macula.

Maculopathy

Disease at the macula is one of the causes of blindness in diabetes. It is usually insidious in its development and visual acuity can be shown to decline over months or even years. It more commonly occurs in NIDD patients than those with IDD. The appearance of hard exudates often in rings, close to the macula, gives warning that the disease may spread on to the macula; when it does so visual acuity falls, usually irreversibly.

Macular oedema

This is a thickening or swelling of the macular portion of the retina. It occurs both in the presence of hard exudates and less commonly in their absence. It is very difficult to visualize by direct ophthalmoscopy; the macular region appears indistinct and has a subtle grey discolouration. Fluorescein angiography reveals extensive capillary leakage. It may progress rapidly so that early recognition and treatment (laser photocoagulation) are required; even then vision is threatened.

Pre-proliferative lesions

Ischaemia of the retina probably predisposes to the development of dangerous formation of new vessels, perhaps in response to an 'angiogenic factor'. Lesions indicating an ischaemic and therefore 'pre-proliferative' retina are:
1   Multiple dot and blot haemorrhages.
2   Cotton wool spots (previously 'soft exudates'); these are small zones of intracellular oedema in the retinal nerve fibre layer developing in an area of ischaemia from capillary closure. They are indistinct, large (disc size) and pale.

3   Venous beading, loops and reduplication (Plate 2).
4   Arterial streaking manifested by parallel white streaks on either side of
the arteries.
5   IRMA (intraretinal microvascular-abnormality) are fine vascular loops
lying within the retina, probably representing true intraretinal neovascularization (Plate 2).
6   Atrophic-looking retina.

Proliferative retinopathy

New vessel formation occurs either on the optic disc (new vessels on the
disc, NVD) or in the periphery of the retina (new vessels elsewhere, NVE)
(Plates 3 and 4). Disc new vessels may grow forward into the vitreous and
the risk of vitreous haemorrhage is very great, resulting in blindness in
about 30% of cases after 3 years if untreated. The hazard is less for
peripheral new vessels (NVE) although they often precede the development
of disc new vessels (NVD).

Large pre-retinal haemorrhages may occur, not always affecting vision,
but vitreous haemorrhages are more serious causing blindness rapidly,
painlessly and without warning. The vitreous usually clears after some
weeks with some recovery of vision, but with repeated haemorrhages vision
deteriorates permanently.

Advanced diabetic eye disease

The development of fibroglial proliferation usually following new vessel
formation and haemorrhage leads to the appearance of white fibrous
strands which contract and cause severe retinal detachment and tears
(Plate 4).

When new vessel formation occurs in the anterior chamber and on the
iris (rubeosis iridis) a particularly painful and intractable form of glaucoma
develops (rubeotic glaucoma). When conservative management for this
condition fails, enucleation is sometimes needed for the relief of pain.

Management of retinopathy and prevention of blindness

Prevention, screening and active treatment for established retinopathy are
the three principal approaches to the management of diabetic retinopathy.

Prevention

The importance of control of diabetes in relation to the development of
retinopathy is described on p. 117. No drug therapy is known to be

successful. Clofibrate does lead to a diminution of exudates but without improvement of vision. The role of aldose reductase inhibitors and somatostatin analogues are under evaluation.

Screening

Screening for retinopathy in order to prevent blindness has become a major part of diabetes care and any system must be carefully organized. It is important because retinopathy needing treatment by photocoagulation must be detected before vision has deteriorated, otherwise improvement is unlikely.

The frequency with which retinal screening is needed must be flexible. An annual examination is recommended, but when retinopathy is established, and especially when pre-proliferative changes are present, or if the macula is threatened, then more frequent examination and collaboration with an ophthalmologist becomes important. The eyes of all new diabetics should be examined at diagnosis, bearing in mind that, especially amongst older patients, up to one-quarter of patients may have changes even at the time of diagnosis of diabetes. Patients with proteinuria have a high risk of developing retinopathy and should be examined more frequently.

VISUAL ACUITY

Facilities for testing visual acuity using a Snellen chart should now be routine in diabetic clinics. The best corrected vision should be recorded, using either the patient's own glasses, or by optical correction using a 'pin-hole' held in front of the eye. Patients whose visual acuity is poor, or those in whom it is found to decline, should be referred to an ophthalmologist for proper diagnosis and treatment.

Collaboration with selected and informed local ophthalmic opticians in some areas can be invaluable; a form of cooperation card recording visual acuity as measured by the optician can be held by the patient and brought to the clinic. Many opticians will also be able to assist by recording the presence of retinopathy.

FUNDUS EXAMINATION

This should be undertaken through dilated pupils in a darkened room, and these facilities must be available in diabetic clinics. Tropicamide (1% Mydriacil) eye drops are the best for dilating the pupils; they have a rapid action and reversal takes place spontaneously and rapidly in 2–3 hours without the need for reversal with pilocarpine eye drops, which in any case do not reverse the effects on accommodation.

Physicians caring for diabetics should be trained to examine fundi properly and be able to detect lesions needing more specialized care from ophthalmologists, and in particular those likely to need laser photocoagulation. It is not practicable for routine screening to be undertaken by ophthalmologists themselves.

RETINAL PHOTOGRAPHY

Screening by retinal photography is gaining popularity. It may be undertaken either by non-mydriatic cameras yielding polaroid prints, or by standard retinal photography through dilated pupils. Several studies have indicated that some lesions, especially fine peripheral new vessels, may be missed by these techniques. Perhaps the best use for retinal photography will be to demonstrate the absence of any retinal lesions; once present specialized examination is needed. Retinal photography cannot replace the need for visual acuity testing or in general for proper fundus examination.

FLUORESCEIN ANGIOGRAPHY

Fluorescein angiography is useful in detecting exudation from intraretinal vascular abnormalities and in detecting areas of ischaemia in the capillary bed, with resulting 'non-perfusion'. It will also confirm the presence of neovascularization if there is any doubt about this. Positive findings may indicate the need for laser therapy. The detection of the source and extent of macular oedema and the extent of areas of non-perfusion are the main indications for fluorescein angiography, because these abnormalities cannot be assessed by ophthalmoscopy. This method of investigation is also useful in cases of unexplained loss of central vision when the shutdown of capillaries or cystic changes at the fovea may be the cause of poor visual acuity.

INDICATIONS FOR REFERRAL TO AN OPHTHALMOLOGIST

These include:
1 Decline of corrected visual acuity from any cause.
2 The presence of pre-proliferative lesions.
3 Proliferative retinopathy with or without vitreous haemorrhage.
4 Lesions which herald the development of maculopathy, especially the appearance of exudates near the macula.

Treatment by laser photocoagulation

The prevention of blindness requires treatment of appropriate lesions by photocoagulation before and vision has deteriorated and before vitreous haemorrhage has occurred (Plates 5 and 6). The indications for this treatment are:

1 New vessels on the optic disc. Peripheral ablative photocoagulation causes regression of these vessels, thus preventing vitreous haemorrhage; treatment should not be delayed. Laser treatment is most effective in this situation, especially if it is undertaken before haemorrhage or any deterioration of vision has occurred.

2 Peripheral new vessels. These are treated directly by laser burns. Treatment is less urgent than for disc new vessels.

3 Exudative retinopathy. These should be treated, especially when circinate exudates develop near the macula. Photocoagulation is indicated when visual acuity begins to deteriorate by one or two lines on the Snellen chart; leaking blood vessels at the centre of the rings of exudate are treated by photocoagulation to prevent further leakage.

4 Maculopathy as described on p. 135.

VITREOUS HAEMORRHAGE

If this occurs vision is temporarily lost, but will improve somewhat as the haemorrhage resorbs. Photocoagulation should be performed after the vitreous has cleared. If bilateral vitreous haemorrhages have occurred, patients should be admitted for complete bed-rest so that vitreous clearing is accelerated and early laser treatment can be performed. If the vitreous becomes permanently opaque after repeated haemorrhages, then vitrectomy can be performed; its success is limited by the existence of retinopathy, but it often helps those who have been completely blind to obtain some navigational vision. The procedure of vitrectomy can also be used to remove some pre-retinal fibroglial membranes and relieve traction detachments of the retina.

The lens: refractive changes and cataract

Refractive changes

The development of myopia (2–3 dioptres) is common in uncontrolled diabetes; it is occasionally the presenting symptom and may be diagnosed as such by an astute optician. This refractive shift is due to osmotic changes in the lens and possibly to factors involving ionic pumps as well. The refractive change is reversed after starting insulin (and much more rarely after starting tablets) and patients become hypermetropic for a time, perhaps 2 or 3 weeks, during which they experience difficulty with reading and their insulin injection technique. They are sometimes alarmed unless warned. The use of temporary glasses at this time is helpful.

The onset of cataract formation is sometimes accompanied by the development of myopia while blurred vision and diplopia are common symptoms during hypoglycaemia.

Cataract

Cataract formation in diabetics is one of the most frequently observed problems and is commoner than in non-diabetics. Cataracts have an increased prevalance in adult diabetics with a 3–4-fold increased risk in the age range 50–64 years, this excess risk decreasing in later years. Activation of the polyol pathway (not necessarily leading to an accumulation of sorbitol) may amplify oxidative mechanisms already important for senile cataract development while glycation or carbamylation of lens proteins could play a further part in the process.

Cataract takes various forms. It can appear as the dots, flakes, spokes or subcapsular opacities ('snowstorm') of cortical cataract; or with nuclear sclerosis in which opacities are dense, central and may have yellow-brown discoloration. The rate of progress of lens opacities is difficult to predict. It is usually slow and, as interference with vision is usually late and treatment often effective, it is justifiable to be reasonably optimistic to the patient. The word 'cataract' may be frightening and is better avoided in describing the minor lens opacities which are so often seen in elderly diabetics.

Juvenile diabetic cataract is a very rare but distinctive form of cataract which develops acutely in young IDD patients. A dense subcapsular or floccular cataract forms at the posterior pole in just a few weeks or months leading to blindness in that eye. It is usually bilateral and irreversible. Its cause is unknown and it is not particularly associated with poor diabetic control.

Treatment for mature cataract is by surgical extraction followed by lens implant, contact lens application or the provision of spectacles. A high success rate is expected, although occasional disappointments occur if extensive retinopathy has been hidden by the presence of the lens opacities.

Glaucoma

Glaucoma occurs in diabetics as in others; evidence of an increased prevalence is weak and a reported association with autonomic neuropathy has not been confirmed. The association of proliferative retinopathy with rubeosis iridis and intractable glaucoma has been discussed on p. 136. The presence of glaucoma usually means that the eyes should not be dilated for retinal examination.

The iris

The iris is occasionally affected in diabetes in several ways:
1   New vessel formation, i.e. rubeosis iridis (p. 136).
2   Reduction in pupillary size and light reaction, especially in relation to autonomic neuropathy (p. 147).
3   Iritis occurs in a small number of patients in relation to autonomic neuropathy (p. 147).
4   Loss of pigment can occur.

Ocular palsies

Acute, reversible ocular palsies, notably of the IIIrd and VIth nerves occur in diabetes as 'mononeuropathies' and are described in detail on p. 155.

The blind diabetic

Blindness may develop suddenly following vitreous haemorrhage from new vessels, or insidiously over weeks or months as exudative maculopathy or macular oedema gradually progress. Rubeotic glaucoma is particularly painful and disagreeable though relatively uncommon. Retinal detachment also occurs and may cause blindness. It also occurs as a result of cataract formation.

Once blind, the patient should register with the local authority because some amenities and a little financial help are available. Rehabilitation is available for suitable patients at the Royal National Institute for the Blind Centre at Torquay. Reading braille is a valuable asset but some diabetics have a subtle sensory neuropathy affecting the fingers which prevents them doing so.

The best techniques for the blind for injecting insulin is the insulin 'pen' equipment described on p. 232. Alternatively fixed pre-set syringes are useful. The 'click–count' syringe in which each palpable 'click' corresponds to two units of insulin are not easy to use.

Urine testing is feasible using equipment which presents the results with an audible signal.

Further reading

Kritzinger E.E. & Taylor K.G. (1984). *Diabetic Eye Disease*. MTP Press, Lancaster

15: Diabetic Neuropathy

Peripheral nerves are prone to damage in patients with diabetes. Nerve function deteriorates in response to pressure, ischaemia or metabolic abnormalities and these are the chief causes of neuropathies in diabetes. Also alcohol, which can itself cause neuropathy, tends to make diabetic neuropathies worse. Different patterns of the neuropathies therefore exist; there are pressure palsies, mononeuropathies (probably ischaemic in origin) and diffuse sensory and autonomic polyneuropathy (probably both metabolic and ischaemic in orgin). Only the latter is related to duration of diabetes, is progressive and occurs in long-term patients often alongside other diabetic complications. Pressure palsies and mononeuropathies are not specific for diabetes, unrelated to duration or other complications, and often recover. Painful neuropathies develop either in association with established neuropathies or independently and are poorly understood. A suggested classification for diabetic neuropathies is shown in Table 15.1.

Pathology

Symmetrical sensory neuropathy

Axon degeneration of both myelinated and unmyelinated fibres is demonstrable, although there is a spectrum of disease ranging from predominantly small fibre loss (representing pain and temperature modalities and autonomic fibres) to a major loss of all fibre types. There is also evidence of axonal regeneration in most nerve biopsies taken from diabetic patients, even when the neuropathy is clinically very mild. Segmental demyelination is commonly observed in nerve biopsies, and the process of remyelination also witnessed.

Vascular changes

Evidence for hypoxia in diabetic nerves is growing. It has been found in experimental diabetic neuropathies as well as by direct *in vivo* measurement in the sural nerve of diabetic patients. Evidence for ischaemia in the aetiology of diabetic neuropathy is also based on visible abnormalities in

Table 15.1 Clinical classification of neuropathy

1 Symmetrical diffuse neuropathy* Somatic sensory neuropathy Autonomic neuropathy
2 Mononeuropathies* Femoral neuropathy (diabetic amyotrophy) Truncal radiculopathies Cranial nerve palsies (III, VI)
3 Pressure palsies+ Carpal tunnel syndrome Ulnar compression Lateral popliteal compression (foot drop)

* Painful neuropathic syndromes may coexist with both major groups of neuropathies
+ Pressure palsies are non-specific to, but commoner in, patients with diabetes

the vasa nervorum, both in perineurial and endoneurial blood vessels. Endothelial proliferation and reduplication of the surrounding basal lamina contribute to narrowing of the lumen and in some instances, microplatelet thrombi and capillary closure have been described. The patchy distribution of myelinated fibre loss in diabetic neuropathy is however similar to that in some hereditary (therefore non-ischaemic) neuropathies, an observation which weakens the case for a vascular basis for the disease.

Sural nerve biopsy changes correlate poorly with clinical findings. Since striking abnormalities are already demonstrable when the clinical neuropathy is very mild, it seems likely that major changes occur before any clinical disease can be detected. Nerve biopsy is a research procedure and is not of diagnostic value in these cases.

The CNS is not normally affected by diabetes, although there are a few reports of degenerative changes. Some of these may be due to a 'dying back' process extending centrally from the peripheral nerves.

Autonomic neuropathy

Most information on autonomic nerves comes from post-mortem examinations, although major degenerative changes have been described in vagi removed during gastric surgery (Fig. 15.1). Autonomic ganglia show degenerative changes, and fibre loss or degeneration have been described in corpora cavernosa of the penis and bladder wall. Inflammatory cellular infiltrates in autonomic tissue (ganglia and nerve bundles of viscera) have been seen in some autopsies from severely affected autonomic neuropathy patients, leading to the suggestion that immunological damage might play some role in the development of this disorder.

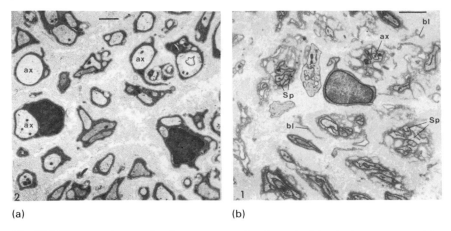

(a)   (b)

Fig. 15.1 Electron micrographs of transverse section through abdominal vagus nerves (a) of a normal subject aged 24 years, showing a dense population of unmyelinated axons (ax); and (b) from a severe autonomic neuropathy patient with intractable gastroparesis aged 28 years showing marked reduction of the axons both in density and size.

Mononeuropathies

Multifocal lesions with patchy fibre loss have been seen in the very rare instances where autopsy examination has been possible. Vascular occlusion may be responsible, but observations are few.

Biochemical changes

Important biochemical changes have been demonstrated in peripheral nerves from diabetic patients as well as animal models. Schwann cells and endoneurial capillaries contain the enzyme aldose reductase which converts glucose to the sugar alcohol sorbitol, which is in turn metabolized to fructose. Thus nerves from diabetics contain increased amounts of glucose, sorbitol and fructose. The accumulation of sorbitol might be responsible for impairment of nerve function and eventually the axon degeneration responsible for neuropathy, although this mechanism has not been established. Aldose reductase inhibitors have been developed during recent years and their effects extensively studied; some functional and biochemical abnormalities, notably sorbitol accumulation, can be restored to normal by their use both in animals and in man. However their effects on the development of neuropathy and its symptoms are still uncertain even though recent serial nerve biopsies suggest that some nerve fibre regeneration may take place.

Myoinositol is an important constituent of cell membrane phospholipids;

it is depleted in peripheral nerves in experimental diabetes and feeding myoinositol to these animals reverses some of the abnormalities. There is no evidence in man that this substance is depleted, nor that supplements have any effect on clinical neuropathy.

Glycation of myelin and other neural constituents is known to occur and may alter their composition so that they are prone to damage probably by immunological mechanisms. These observations are preliminary.

Electrophysiology

Electrophysiological abnormalities occur very frequently in long-standing diabetics whether or not symptoms are present and, conversely, those with the most severe symptomatic painful neuropathies may prove to have almost no electrophysiological changes. The value of these tests in practice is therefore very limited; their chief use is in the diagnosis of mono-neuropathies and their distinction from nerve root compressive lesions which require further investigation and treatment.

Electrophysiological abnormalities are numerous. Motor nerve conduction is often moderately reduced, although this observation may be the least relevant in diabetic neuropathy which is predominantly sensory. Sensory conduction and amplitude of evoked responses are helpful tests, while measurement of F-wave latencies may in some instances provide the most sensitive test. Recording from single nerve fibres is now possible and by this technique absence of peripheral sympathetic nerve fibres has been shown to occur more frequently in diabetic neuropathies than in others.

Clinical description of the neuropathies

Distal symmetrical sensory and autonomic neuropathy

This is the commonest form of diabetic neuropathy and is associated with autonomic neuropathy (Table 15.1). Detectable neuropathy increases as duration of diabetes lengthens; it occurs independently of other diabetic complications but in longstanding diabetics is often associated with them. It is permanent and irreversible. Its severity varies greatly from one patient to another and as with other complications some are spared altogether.

The neuropathy is symmetrical affecting the feet in a stocking distribution, with rare symptomatic involvement of the hands in which symptoms are more commonly due to carpal tunnel compression. It is predominantly a sensory neuropathy in which small nerve fibres carrying pain, temperature and autonomic modalities are affected first. As the disease advances, all fibre types are affected.

The neuropathy is often symptomless and this is the chief hazard to the

Table 15.2 Clinical features of sensory neuropathy

Symptomless
Paraesthesiae
Painful syndrome
Numbness
Sensation of coldness
Neuropathic ulceration
Charcot joints

unwary patient. Later patients may be aware of numbness; sensations of coldness and paraesthesiae are common (Table 15.2). The disorder sometimes worsens until rarely there is almost complete anaesthesia below the knees. Severe pain of the type described on p. 153 is occasionally the predominant feature. The most serious consequence of diabetic neuropathy is development of diabetic foot problems (see p. 172).

DIAGNOSIS AND EVALUATION

Careful examination is needed to detect diabetic neuropathy. Non-diabetic causes must always be considered and investigated when appropriate. Motor weakness is very uncommon and sensory abnormalities can be difficult to detect at the bed-side. Ankle reflexes are usually absent, while the knee jerks are retained till an advanced stage. Pain and temperature modalities of sensation are lost first and thus surprisingly severe lesions of the feet may be seen while light touch sensation remains grossly intact. Eventually all sensory modalities can be affected.

Sophisticated techniques are not normally needed for investigation. EMG examination rarely helps in symmetrical neuropathy beyond establishing the presence of neuropathy, but in the mononeuropathies it is of value in localizing the lesion. Evaluation of vibration perception threshold using a biothesiometer is helpful and recommended (see p. 235) but other tests of sensory function are complex and not suitable for routine clinical use.

NEUROPATHY AND THE HANDS

Diabetic neuropathy rarely causes symptoms in the hands and, when it does, the disease is already advanced in the feet and legs. Numbness and clumsiness of the fingers are unusual and generally due to some other neurological disorder, although impairment of sensation is often sufficient to prevent blind diabetics from reading Braille. Some patients cultivate longer nails in order to increase tactile sensitivity.

Paraesthesiae and numbness in the fingers especially at night are sometimes due to carpal tunnel syndrome, which is easy to diagnose and treat by minor surgery under local anaesthetic.

Interosseous muscle wasting is not uncommon and due to ulnar nerve compression at the elbow; it is accompanied by typical sensory defects in the fourth and fifth fingers. Disability is unusual and there is no satisfactory treatment beyond the advice not to lean on the elbows.

Autonomic neuropathy

Autonomic defects are very common in long-standing diabetics but only rarely cause the unpleasant clinical symptoms described below (Table 15.3). Even when they do occur, these symptoms are often curiously intermittent, though they continue over many years and rarely remit completely. Sympathetic damage also causes major changes of blood flow which may be related to some of the foot problems experienced by diabetics and these are described on p. 174.

We have described a very striking syndrome in which younger IDD patients develop iritis accompanied by severe 'small fibre' neuropathy causing symptomatic autonomic neuropathy, Charcot joints and foot ulcers with arterial calcification in the feet (see p. 176). The mechanisms underlying the association remain to be elucidated.

Table 15.3 Clinical features of autonomic neuropathy

	Clinical syndromes	Other abnormalities	
Cardiovascular:	Postural hypotension Tachycardia		
Sweating:	Gustatory sweating		
Genitourinary:	Impotence Neurogenic bladder		
Gastrointestinal:	Diarrhoea Gastroparesis	Oesophageal mobility Gall bladder emptying	
Respiratory:	Arrests ?Sudden death	?Sleep apnoea Cough reflex	
Eye:		Pupillary responses Pupillary size	} all reduced
Neuro-endocrine responses:		Catecholamines Glucagon Pancreatic polypeptide	

Autonomic neuropathy progresses very slowly; when it is associated with postural hypotension then mortality is increased and sudden unexplained deaths have been reported in a few cases. The development of nephropathy in these patients is not uncommon and deaths then are usually from renal failure.

DIARRHOEA

This is often a catastrophic watery diarrhoea with severe nocturnal exacerbations and faecal incontinence, preceded by abdominal rumblings. Steatorrhoea is not normally a feature. The symptoms are intermittent with normal bowel action or even constipation between bouts. They continue over many years and complete remissions are unusual. Persistent and intractable diarrhoea is also very rare. The diagnosis is made not only by establishing the presence of autonomic neuropathy but it is also absolutely essential to exclude other causes of diarrhoea such as coeliac or pancreatic disease. The diarrhoea is treated with any anti-diarrhoea agent, the best of which is codeine phosphate. Tetracycline in two or three doses of 250 mg has a dramatic effect in about half the cases and should be used at the onset of the attack. The use of clonidine has been described but its efficacy not confirmed.

GASTROPARESIS

Diminished gastric motility and delayed stomach emptying occur sometimes in diabetics with autonomic neuropathy but symptoms are rare. Intermittent vomiting may occur and is very rarely intractable. Diagnosis is established by the presence of a gastric splash and screening during barium studies which show food residue, loss of peristalsis and failure to empty. Endoscopy is needed to exclude other gastric disorders. Complex studies of gastric emptying are helpful but not generally available. Metoclopramide and domperidone are useful in treatment. Most episodes remit and the need for gastric surgery is very rare and not always satisfactory.

POSTURAL HYPOTENSION

This is defined by a postural fall of systolic pressure on standing of more than 30 mm Hg; blood pressure may fall continuously for up to 3 or 4 minutes. The postural fall is very variable and is exacerbated by insulin (Fig. 15.2). Symptoms, which are rare, are also very variable in their severity. Disabling postural hypotension is very uncommon indeed and management is not simple. Patients should stop any medication which aggravates hypotension, notably tranquillizers, anti-depressants and diuretics; they

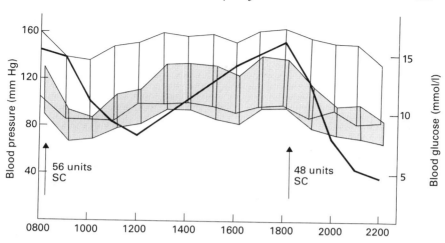

Fig. 15.2 Fluctuations in postural hypotension in relation to subcutaneous (SC) insulin injections. Plain area shows recumbent blood pressure and that on standing is shown in the hatched area.

should sleep with the head of the bed elevated and wear full length elastic stockings. The most effective measures aim to increase blood volume and include a high salt intake and fludrocortisone, using increasing doses up to 0.4 mg daily. Failures are common, and the oedema which results from treatment is often unacceptable. Many other agents have been tried and include combinations of fludrocortisone with flurbiprofen and ephedrine, pindolol and the use of the alpha-agonist midodrine.

RESPIRATORY ARRESTS

Transient respiratory arrests occur sometimes if susceptible neuropathic patients are given agents which depress respiration, notably powerful analgesics and anaesthetics. These patients should be monitored carefully even during minor surgery. It is very likely that some sudden unexpected and unexplained deaths amongst these patients are due to respiratory arrests.

GUSTATORY SWEATING

Facial sweating (including scalp, neck and shoulders) which occurs while eating tasty foods, notably cheese, is a common symptom of autonomic neuropathy (Fig. 15.3). In severe cases the sweat pours down the neck and chest, and sufferers feel they are in a Turkish bath. This symptom provides clinical evidence for the presence of autonomic neuropathy. Some patients

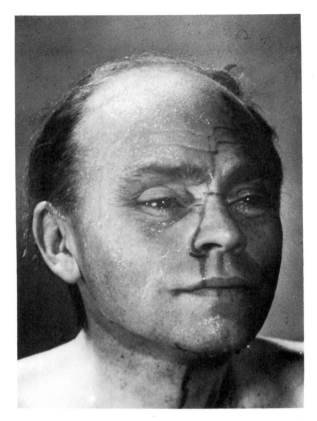

Fig. 15.3 Gustatory sweating in a severe autonomic neuropathy patient, shown a few seconds after chewing cheese. The dark line is from application of starch-iodide powder.

seek treatment which is effected either by avoiding the offending foodstuffs or by the use of anticholinergic agents. The best treatment is with poldine methylsulphate (Nacton) given before each meal; side effects sometimes prove to be unacceptable.

NEUROGENIC BLADDER

Urinary retention is a serious and usually late complication of autonomic neuropathy. It develops following both loss of the normal sensation of bladder distension and failure of detrusor activity. Inadequate micturition and later gross bladder distension occur and may mimic prostatic obstruction; rarely hydronephrosis develops. Persistent urinary tract infections also occur. Treatment includes regular voiding helped by straining and abdominal pressure; the use of cholinergic drugs such as bethanecol, bladder neck dilation, and eventually catheterisation. Careful resection of the bladder neck may help if other measures have failed.

IMPOTENCE

Impotence is a common symptom especially in diabetic men over 55 years of age. It occurs more often in diabetic men than in non-diabetics: about half of diabetics over 55 years of age may be affected while younger patients in their third and fourth decades sometimes have this problem. While neuropathy plays an important role, vascular and psychogenic causes are also relevant and the whole subject is discussed below.

Diagnosis of autonomic neuropathy

Autonomic dysfunction is common in both longstanding and older diabetics and its presence is easily confirmed by simple bedside tests described below. Symptoms from autonomic neuropathy are much less common and, before they are attributed to autonomic neuropathy (which must of course be shown to be present), other disorders must be excluded if serious errors are to be avoided.

Clinical indicators of autonomic neuropathy include the presence of gustatory sweating, a resting tachycardia, postural hypotension and rarely a gastric splash.

The following bedside tests of autonomic function are valuable; normal and abnormal values are shown in Table 15.4.

HEART RATE VARIATION ON DEEP BREATHING

The normal acceleration and deceleration of heart rate during respiration (sinus arrythmia) is reduced early in the course of autonomic neuropathy due to cardiac vagal denervation; this phenomenon provides the basis for

Table 15.4 Normal values for autonomic function tests*

	Normal	Abnormal
Heart rate variation (deep breathing)	>15	<10
Heart rate on standing (at 15 seconds)	>15	<12
Heart rate on standing 30 : 15 ratio	>1.04	<1.00
Valsalva ratio	>1.21	<1.20
Postural systolic pressure fall at 2 min	<10 mmHg	>30 mmHg

* These tests decline with age. The figures given here apply generally in those less than 60 years old.

Chapter 15

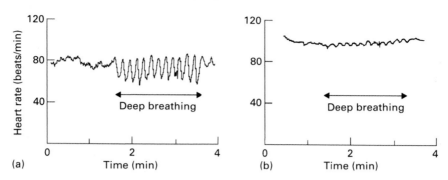

Fig. 15.4 Heart rate variation at rest and during deep breathing (a) in a normal subject and (b) in a patient with severe autonomic neuropathy. Normally the heart rate accelerates and decelerates with inspiration and expiration respectively; these changes are reduced or absent in autonomic neuropathy.

the simplest and most sensitive test for the presence of autonomic neuropathy. Heart rate is increased during deep breathing at a rate of 6 breaths per minute (5 seconds in and 5 seconds out). The average heart rate difference (maximum minus minimum at the end of each breath) over 5 breaths is recorded. While the use of a heart rate monitor is the simplest method of conducting this test, an ordinary electrocardiograph can be used (Fig. 15.4).

HEART RATE INCREASE ON STANDING

On standing up there is an immediate and rapid increase in heart rate which overshoots the eventual rate on standing, which is higher than that when lying down. Absence of this overshoot is evidence of a cardiac vagal defect (Fig. 15.5).

The actual heart rate increase is recorded at the peak of the overshoot or if there is no overshoot, 15 seconds after standing up. An alternative index is the 30:15 ratio which records the ratio of the R:R interval of the 30th in relation to the 15th beat after standing.

VALSALVA MANOEUVRE

This is performed by asking the patient to blow into the empty barrel of a 20 ml syringe attached to a mercury sphygnomanometer; a pressure of 40 mmHg should be maintained for 10 seconds. The ratio of the maximum heart rate during blowing to the minimum (bradycardia) after cessation is recorded. The test should not be performed on patients with proliferative retinopathy.

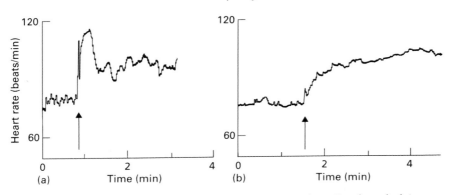

Fig. 15.5 Heart rate changes on standing; normally the effect of standing from the lying position is to cause an overshoot of heart rate (a) an effect which is lost in autonomic neuropathy (b) together with a progressive reduction in the cardiac acceleration at 15 seconds.

BLOOD PRESSURE CHANGE ON STANDING

A decrease of more than 30 mmHg systolic pressure is abnormal. Patients should remain standing for at least 3 minutes during which the systolic pressure may continue to fall.

Painful neuropathy

Disabling pain as opposed to discomfort from paraesthesiae is an uncommon symptom of diabetic neuropathy. It is to be expected in the thigh in patients with proximal motor neuropathy, over the abdomen or chest in cases of truncal radiculopathy or in the feet and legs if it occurs in symmetrical peripheral neuropathy. The pain causes exceptional distress because it is protracted and unremitting and may last several months or sometimes longer. Constant burning sensations, likened sometimes to walking on burning sand, paraesthesiae and shooting or searing pains are often described. There is a subjective sensation of swollen feet. A highly characteristic feature is that of exquisite sensitivity and discomfort to contact with clothes and bed clothes. The symptoms are worse at night causing insomnia and depression, and profound weight loss is usual, often leading to a fruitless search for malignant conditions. Sensory loss is distal, usually less extensive than the pains, and sometimes negligible; thus painful symmetrical neuropathy can occur in the initial absence of sensory signs or electrophysiological changes, or it may accompany severe neuropathic features in which the numb foot is exquisitely painful (the 'painless painful foot'). Patients are so distressed that they may seek several opinions on their condition.

TREATMENT

Treatment of painful neuropathy is always difficult; above all, the promise of eventual remission of the severest symptoms is needed to sustain patients during the worst months of their illness. Diabetic control should be optimal, using insulin if necessary. Regular analgesics are essential, although drugs of addiction should be avoided except possibly to help sleep during the worst period of the illness. Tricyclic antidepressants help to alleviate insomnia and depression and may also have a specific and beneficial effect on this type of pain. Amitriptyline or nortriptyline are used, the latter in a useful combination with fluphenazine (Motival). Carbamazepine and mexiletine may help. The use of a cutaneous nerve stimulator at sites of pain is sometimes helpful to morale.

The most severe and unpleasant symptoms of painful neuropathy resolve in 6–8 months, occasionally up to 1 or even 2 years. The symptoms may disappear completely and leave no residual signs. When the features are less dramatic, some discomfort and paraesthesiae may persist for years though normal body weight is always restored. Relapses are very uncommon indeed.

Mononeuropathies

Single nerves, or groups of nerve roots, are affected. The rapid onset, severity and eventual recovery of these lesions are in striking contrast to the gradually progressive development of diffuse sensory and autonomic neuropathy. The lesions can occur at any age or duration of diabetes, although they are commoner in older patients, and they are unrelated to other diabetic complications. It is always important to exclude other causes of nerve or nerve root compression in these cases.

PROXIMAL MOTOR NEUROPATHY (FEMORAL NEUROPATHY)

Pain with or without wasting of one, or sometimes both, thighs is the cardinal feature of this condition. The quality of the continuous pain which affects the thigh and may extend medially below the knee is identical to that described on p. 153. It may cause insomnia and sometimes profound weight loss. The weakness is sometimes sufficiently severe to cause the knee to give way and patients may fall. Examination always shows wasting and weakness of the quadriceps, and usually of the iliopsoas and thigh adductors (innervated by the obturator nerve) as well. The knee jerk is absent, while the ankle jerk may be intact. Diagnosis must be confirmed by careful clinical examination and needs electrophysiological confirmation. It is essential to exclude nerve root compression. Lumbar spine X-ray should be taken and sometimes myelography or magnetic resonance imaging is needed as well. CSF proteins are often raised in this condition and may be 1000 mg/l or more.

Recovery is the rule, between 6 and 12 months after the onset. Principles of management are described on p. 154.

TRUNCAL RADICULOPATHIES

Characteristic pain affects areas of the trunk, more commonly abdominal than thoracic, in the distribution of groups of nerve roots either unilaterally or bilaterally. It can encircle the trunk in nerve root distribution resembling root compression from which it must be distinguished. On very rare occasions motor weakness and abdominal wall muscles cause a striking bulging to occur. Recovery is expected in less than 12 months, severe symptoms rarely persisting for more than 2 years.

CRANIAL NERVE PALSIES

Ocular palsies are more common in the diabetics than non-diabetics. Patients tend to be older and the aetiology is thought to be vascular. The cranial nerves most affected are the third and the sixth. The evidence for an association of seventh nerve palsy with diabetes is very weak.

The onset of diplopia is abrupt and, in third nerve palsy, it is often preceded by some pain behind or just above the eye. The pupil is usually spared, and ptosis is very uncommon. Recovery takes place in 3 months and relapse is very unusual.

Pressure palsies

Carpal tunnel syndrome is commoner in diabetics than non-diabetics (see p. 147). Ulnar nerve compression at the elbow probably occurs more often in diabetics than others, causing numbness of the fourth and fifth fingers and wasting of the interossei.

Foot drop results either from pressure on the lateral popliteal nerve at the knee or from L5/S1 nerve root lesions; it is uncertain whether these problems are related to diabetes. Nerve root lesions require correct diagnosis and treatment in their own right while patients with lateral popliteal lesions sometimes, but not always, recover spontaneously.

Impotence

The development of impotence has four major causes, apart from a reversible impotence which may develop in almost any state of ill health. It may be psychogenic, which is probably the commonest single cause; it is sometimes neurogenic in origin, occasionally due to vascular disease (poor arterial inflow or increased venous leak from the penis), or it can have an endocrine basis. Only neurogenic impotence is specific to diabetes; it does not have an endocrine basis and gonadotrophins and testosterone levels are normal in diabetic patients.

Neuropathic impotence develops in relation to other diabetic complications and it is more likely to be present when there is evidence of both somatic and autonomic neuropathy. It is by no means always present even in patients with severe neuropathy and, conversely, it is sometimes the earliest symptom of neuropathy when there are few other features.

Once present, neuropathic impotence is permanent and irreversible. Its onset is always gradual and slowly progressive over months or years. Erectile ability fails first at a time when ejaculation is retained. Retrograde ejaculation sometimes occurs. Nocturnal erections are absent in these patients whereas they are often retained in psychogenic impotence. Libido is normal. It is important to distinguish neurogenic from psychogenic impotence wherever possible, although this is often difficult. Psychogenic impotence presents in some contrasting ways; it is often abrupt in its onset sometimes in response to adverse circumstances, nocturnal erections often persist and the condition is intermittent and potentially reversible.

Diagnosis

A careful history helps to distinguish organic from psychogenic impotence. Drug-induced impotence, especially from hypotensive agents, should be excluded.

Physical assessment should include examination of the genitalia; endocrine referral is required if there is evidence of hypogonadism. Neurological examination is needed to determine the presence of somatic and autonomic neuropathy. Abnormal autonomic function tests provide some guidance in diagnosis but do not alone establish the presence of neuropathic impotence.

Nocturnal penile tumescence can be measured with relatively simple apparatus; its preservation points to a psychogenic cause for impotence, although this test does not indicate whether satisfactory penile rigidity is achieved.

Penile injection of papaverine into the corpus cavernosum is the simplest method of excluding a vascular cause for impotence; satisfactory erection occurs even when neuropathy is present but not if the cause is vascular. Penile blood pressure can also be assessed by Doppler probes. More complex assessment by penile perfusion cavernometry is undertaken in specialist centres to identify the exact vascular cause for impotence.

The rare endocrine causes of impotence are excluded by measurement of testosterone, prolactin and gonadotrophins.

Management

Counselling of husband and wife is almost always needed, especially if the impotence is psychogenic in origin. Neuropathic impotence is however permanent and there is no cure. Patients and their spouses need to understand this to eliminate suspicion and mistrust. This proper explanation suffices for many couples and they often seek no further treatment. Androgen treatment is contraindicated because it merely serves to increase libido without restoring potency.

For patients requiring active treatment, there are now several options available, although none of these is entirely satisfactory.

1 Erection can be induced by application of a partial vacuum to the penis after venous occlusion. This is applied with a specially designed re-usable condom with a vacuum pump attached. It is non-invasive, but the apparatus is cumbersome and relatively expensive (see p. 235).

2 Papaverine (40–80 mg) can be injected directly into the corpus cavernosum. This treatment has some obvious drawbacks: protracted erections, sepsis and penile fibrosis can result in the long-term.

3 A surgical prosthesis can be inserted. The simplest technique is the insertion of a malleable silastic rod which is often effective especially when ejaculation is retained. More elaborate inflatable prostheses can be inserted but the apparatus is more complex, prone to failure and very expensive. Few centres have much experience.

Further reading

Bannister R. (ed) (1988). *Autonomic Failure*. Oxford University Press, Oxford
Dyck P.J., Thomas P.K., Asbury A.K., Winegrad A.I. & Port D. (1987). *Diabetic Neuropathy*. W.B. Saunders Company, London

16: Cardiovascular Disease in Diabetes

Introduction

Cardiovascular disease is the major cause of death in patients with both IDD and NIDD. This chapter will consider the problems outlined in Table 16.1, except for peripheral vascular disease which is covered in Chapter 17.

Table 16.1 Cardiovascular diseases occurring in excess in diabetes

Ischaemic heart disease (coronary artery disease)
Angina
Myocardial infarct
Left ventricular and congestive cardiac failure
Hypertension
Conduction defects
A specific diabetic cardiomyopathy?
Cerebrovascular disease
Stroke
Peripheral vascular disease

Extent of the problem

NON-INSULIN-DEPENDENT DIABETES

Epidemiological studies of the mortality of patients with NIDD in Western populations almost all show very considerable increases in mortality from cardiovascular disease, especially coronary artery disease, when compared with age-matched non-diabetic subjects. Overall 50–65% of all deaths in these patients are from cardiovascular causes. The mortality ratio for diabetics : non-diabetics varies from about 1.5 up to 4. Relative risk ratios are usually higher for younger patients especially younger women. While the mortality from coronary artery disease in the non-diabetic population of the USA has fallen by over 20% in the past 20 years, this fall has not been apparent among diabetics. This huge cardiovascular risk is however not inevitable — in Japan, coronary artery disease accounts for less than 7% of diabetic deaths. This protection is lost by Japanese migrants to Hawaii, suggesting that environmental rather than genetic factors are most important. Differing cholesterol levels provide one possible explanation.

158

INSULIN-DEPENDENT DIABETES

Cardiovascular mortality in IDD is strongly related to the presence of persistent proteinuria, and thus to diabetic renal disease. For these patients the overall relative cardiovascular mortality is 40 times that of the non-diabetic population while the rate for those without persistent proteinuria is about four-fold (Fig. 16.1). Women have a further two-fold increase in relative mortality, but the excess risk in both sexes decreases with increasing age. About 60% of those with proteinuria die of cardiovascular disease rather than renal failure, and this figure has probably increased since the availability of renal transplantation and chronic ambulatory peritoneal dialysis (CAPD).

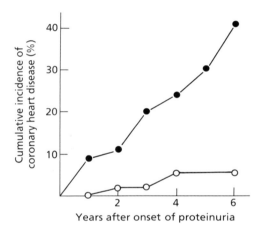

Fig. 16.1 Relative mortality of patients with IDD with (•—•) and without (○—○) persistent proteinuria, compared with the non-diabetic population (from Jensen, T. *et al.* (1987). coronary heart disease in Type 1 diabetes. *Diabetologia*, **30**, 144–148).

Pathology

Most post-mortem studies of coronary artery disease show an increase in atherosclerosis among diabetic subjects compared with non-diabetics, with a suggestion that the diabetics had more diffuse disease and more previous myocardial infarcts; the same has been found based on ECG changes. However the duration of diabetes has not been closely related to the amount of coronary disease in most cases. Whether the greater prevalence of cardiac failure in diabetes is related to more extensive ischaemic heart disease, to the greater number of infarcts sustained or to a specific diabetic cardiomyopathy remains controversial. In practical terms the distinction is of little relevance.

Clinical description

Coronary artery disease may cause sudden death or present with angina pectoris, myocardial infarction and, less often, with unexplained left ventricular failure. In general the investigation and management of these syndromes is exactly the same in the diabetic as in the non-diabetic, although there are several clinical features of note. The whole patient must be assessed; it is of little value performing a CABG to relieve angina if the patient remains crippled by claudication.

Angina pectoris

Angina is more common in diabetics but the clinical presentation is similar. Electrocardiographic evidence of ST depression or T-wave inversion are found more often in diabetics than in normoglycaemic subjects, and mild ST segment depression and T-wave inversion can be induced following glucose loading. Exercise testing and thallium scans are used along conventional lines.

TREATMENT OF ANGINA

Nitrates, beta-blockers, calcium antagonists and aspirin are all suitable for use in diabetics, though negatively inotropic agents should be avoided wherever possible if there is any suggestion of heart failure (more common in diabetes). We use specific beta-1 beta-blockers such as atenolol and metoprolol with success in insulin-treated patients though some physicians still avoid them because of the small but real risk of loss of hypoglycaemic warning symptoms and slow recovery.

The investigation of choice for severe angina unresponsive to medical treatment, for those with evidence of severe multi-vessel disease and those with angina following infarction is coronary angiography. The mortality risk is less than 0.1%. Diffuse coronary heart disease, as found by angiography and precluding possible revascularization, is probably no commoner in diabetics and occurs in less than 10% of the cases.

Coronary artery bypass graft (CABG) was initially associated with higher mortality rates than in non-diabetics, though operative mortality is now less than 5% in those patients with good left ventricular function. Coronary angioplasty is a promising technique but its place in the diabetic is not yet final. Criteria should, at present, be those used in the non-diabetic.

Myocardial infarction

Both IDD and NIDD patients are at high risk from myocardial infarction.

Mortality both in hospital and during the first month is approximately doubled from 15–20% in the non-diabetic to 25–40%, and the trend continues for the next 1 or 2 years. The mortality is not due to larger infarcts and the majority of deaths are caused by pump failure.

Clinically myocardial infarction sometimes presents with little or no chest pain, and this is possibly more common in diabetics. Other presentations are unexplained heart failure, uncontrolled diabetes, vomiting, confusion or collapse. Any diabetic with these symptoms or with other unexplained illness must have a full 12-lead ECG performed.

Whether the achievement of excellent diabetic control during the period after infarction is of benefit is controversial. We treat such patients with an insulin pump or by glucose insulin infusions aiming to keep blood glucose between 4 and 10 mmol/l. Details are the same as those for surgery (p. 107), although higher doses of insulin are usually needed, presumably reflecting the stress hormone responses of cortisol, catecholamines and glucagon. The blood glucose on admission is an indicator of outcome, levels above 20 mmol/l being associated with a very high mortality — this probably reflects the size of the infarct rather than an effect of preceding diabetic control.

THROMBOLYTIC AGENTS AND ASPIRIN

The benefit of aspirin and streptokinase, tissue plasminogin activator and APSAC have been described recently. Their place is not well-defined and no studies have been reported in diabetic subjects.

There are, however, ho specific diabetic contraindications and they should be used along conventional lines.

POST-INFARCT TREATMENT

Use of beta-blockers for 1–2 years following infarction may reduce total mortality among diabetics though many patients with established or incipient heart failure cannot be treated. Any such patient should be energetically treated for heart failure, probably including an angiotensin converting enzyme (ACE) inhibitor in the regime.

Conduction disorders

Diabetics with autonomic neuropathy have increased resting heart rates both during the day and during sleep, as a result of impaired vagal function. Otherwise, amongst fit diabetics, there is no evidence of any excess of cardiac rhythm disorders, but first-degree heart block and right bundle branch block are probably more common. Patients requiring permanent pacemakers for complete heart block and sick sinus syndrome are over-represented by diabetics. Management should be along identical lines to the non-diabetic.

A recent suggestion that QT intervals are prolonged in diabetic patients, possibly related to autonomic neuropathy, may render them more susceptible to ventricular arrythmias. This may at least partly explain the reported high incidence of sudden death in these patients, most notably during anaesthesia.

Cerebrovascular disease

Cerebrovascular accidents are approximately twice as common in the diabetic population as in the non-diabetic, and mortality of acute stroke is approximately doubled both for those with known and previously undiagnosed diabetes. As with myocardial infarction, there is no good evidence as to whether good diabetic control in the hours and days after a cerebrovascular accident is associated with any improvement in the prognosis for life or functional recovery.

Pathogenesis of cardiovascular disease

The risk factors for vascular disease in diabetics are essentially the same as those in non-diabetics, but even when they are taken together they are insufficient to explain the considerable excess mortality. In NIDD, the presence of several factors may produce a greater risk than simple addition or multiplication of the individual risks would suggest.

The major known factors in the pathogenesis of vascular disease in diabetes are hypertension, hyperlipidaemia and smoking which will be discussed below.

Insulin-dependent diabetes

Proteinuria is the greatest risk factor for patients with IDD, but the relative risk for patients without proteinuria is still increased 4-fold. Blood pressure and lipids are mildly elevated in these patients.

Other areas currently under investigation include the role of fibrinogen and platelet abnormalities, but no definite evidence exists at present.

Non-insulin-dependent diabetes and impaired glucose tolerance

The situation in NIDD is even more complex. Several epidemiological studies, notably those from Bedford and Whitehall, have shown that the increased rates of cardiovascular and cerebrovascular disease apply not only

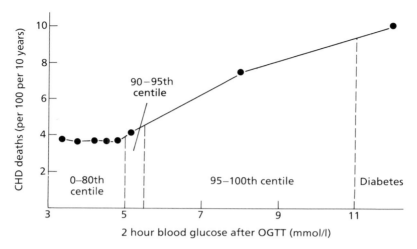

Fig. 16.2 Relationship of coronary heart disease mortality to 2 hour blood glucose after OGTT in the Whitehall study (from Fuller J.H. *et al.* (1983). *British Medical Journal*, **287**, 867–870. CHD, coronary heart disease; OGTT, oral glucose tolerance test).

to those with true diabetes but also to those subjects with impaired glucose tolerance, with 2 hour oral glucose tolerance values of 8–11 mmol/l (capillary) (Fig. 16.2). Thus macrovascular disease is increased among subjects with IGT while microvascular disease only occurs in those with true diabetes, presumably needing a higher threshold glucose level.

The position is made still more complex by the frequent occurrence of obesity in most subjects with NIDD. Glucose tolerance, obesity and hyperlipidaemia are all closely interconnected and it is difficult to establish the role of each alone. Thus, weight loss with no other alteration will improve both glucose tolerance and the lipid profile. The absence of any clear relationship between diabetes duration and cardiovascular risk has led many to propose that they are associated diseases rather than bearing any causal relationship.

Hypertension

Introduction

More diabetics have hypertension than would be expected by chance alone. The reasons for this are not entirely known and are quite complex; the situations in IDD and NIDD are different (Table 16.2). A small number of cases are caused by secondary hypertension of renal, endocrine or drug origin.

Table 16.2 Causes of hypertension in diabetes

Insulin-dependent diabetes
Diabetic nephropathy
Coincidental essential hypertension
Isolated systolic hypertension (usually in arteriopaths)

Non-insulin-dependent diabetes
Diabetic nephropathy
Hypertension of obesity
Coincidental essential hypertension
Isolated systolic hypertension (usually elderly)

Secondary diabetes and hypertension
Acromegaly
Phaeochromocytoma
Cushing's syndrome
Drug-induced (e.g. oestrogens, steroids)

Coincidental secondary hypertension with unrelated diabetes

Table 16.3 WHO criteria for hypertension

	Systolic blood pressure (mmHg)	Diastolic blood pressure (mmHg)
Normotension	< 140	< 90
Borderline	140–159	90–94
Hypertension	⩾ 160	⩾ 95

Criteria for hypertension are shown in Table 16.3.

Blood pressure in all populations, including the diabetic, is one of the strongest risk factors for mortality, though only for cerebrovascular disease, hypertensive renal disease and cardiac failure has anti-hypertensive therapy been shown to reduce mortality. There is no convincing evidence of reduced mortality or morbidity from coronary artery disease in diabetic or non-diabetic groups from anti-hypertensive treatment.

Among diabetic populations, studies from Framingham, Bedford and Whitehall have all shown relationships between blood pressure and cardiovascular mortality; systolic pressure has usually demonstrated a closer correlation than diastolic.

Mechanisms of increased blood pressure

Increased blood pressure in the nephropathic patient, IDD or NIDD, appears to be largely due to sodium retention, possibly related to increased renin secretion from an ischaemic kidney.

The mechanism for most patients with NIDD is less clear. While obesity and hypertension are closely related and appear to have both neurological (sympathetic) and endocrine (renin–angiotensin, catecholamine) components, insulin is also closely related to both and itself has sodium retaining properties. Many have suggested that a single central nervous system defect predisposing to obesity, hypertension, diabetes and possibly atheroma may exist — if so, it remains undiscovered.

Clinical management and investigation

Hypertension has no direct symptoms and most cases are detected during routine examinations or when complications develop (e.g. coronary artery disease or stroke); annual blood pressure checks are recommended for all diabetics, and especially those with any evidence of vascular disease or other risk factors (e.g. proteinuria, smoking, hyperlipidaemia). The possibility of a secondary cause for the hypertension should be considered — there are usually clinical signs or simple clues such as proteinuria.

At least three separate readings should be taken before any treatment is started unless the hypertension is severe or there is definite evidence of end-organ damage (e.g. heart failure). Large cuffs must be used for obese patients or artificially high pressures will be recorded.

All patients should have basic investigations including plasma/serum creatinine and electrolytes and urinalysis; most should have electrocardiograms and a chest X-ray. The need for more extensive studies may then become apparent on the same indications as for non-diabetics.

Other risk factors such as smoking and the lipid profile (see below) should also be considered; the aim of therapy is to reduce the patient's overall risk for cardiovascular disease.

Treatment

Treatment of those patients with nephropathy as a cause of their hypertension has already been discussed in Chapter 13.

NON-DRUG MEASURES

For those without nephropathy the indications for treatment should be the same as for the non-diabetic, that is pressures above 160/95 mmHg for most adults. Initial therapy should always include non-pharmacological methods (Table 16.4) though immediate drug treatment may be needed if hypertension is severe. Weight loss is of particular benefit to both the hypertension and the diabetes while the other changes in lifestyle (smoking, alcohol, exercise) are of wider value.

Table 16.4 Non-drug treatment for hypertension

Weight loss
Reduction of alcohol
Dietary sodium restriction
Dietary potassium increase
Increased dietary fibre
Reduction of simultaneous smoking/caffeine intake
Increased physical exercise

DRUG THERAPY

Most anti-hypertensive agents have significant limitations when given to diabetic patients, either because of metabolic changes they induce, such as worsened glucose tolerance or increased lipids, or because their side-effects are particularly relevant to the diabetic, such as impotence or worsened claudication. The problems of special relevance to diabetes are listed in Table 16.5.

CHOICE OF THERAPY

No rules are possible and the drugs must be chosen to suit the individual patient. As single agents, cardioselective beta-blockers, calcium antagonist, low-dose thiazide diuretics and angiotensin converting enzyme inhibitors are all reasonable choices but a few guidelines can be given:

1 Patients with coronary artery disease should, wherever possible, receive either a beta-blocker or a calcium antagonist as part of their therapy.

2 Those with heart failure require diuretics; the combination with ACE inhibitors is particularly valuable.

3 Beta-blockers should be avoided in those with claudication.

4 Afro-Caribbean patients respond better to diuretics and calcium antagonists than to beta-blockers or ACE inhibitors as single agents.

It is mandatory to ensure at follow-up that these drugs are well-tolerated, including a specific enquiry about impotence in men. Renal function and electrolytes should also be repeated while on therapy with ACE inhibitors and diuretics.

An approximate 'target pressure' should be set — for young people and those with nephropathy this might be as low as 135/80 mmHg while 140/90 would represent good control for most and 160/95 and slightly higher readings mght be acceptable in the elderly; adequate control of systolic pressure is often more difficult to achieve without an excessive fall in diastolic pressure.

Table 16.5 The use of anti-hypertensive drugs in diabetes

Group of drugs	Side effects
Angiotensin-converting enzyme inhibitors	
Captopril	Renal impairment
Enalapril	Hyperkalaemia
Lisinopril	
Calcium antagonists	
Nifedipine	Negative inotropic action
Diltiazem	Ankle oedema
Verapamil	
Cardioselective beta-blockers	
Atenolol	Impairment of glucose tolerance
Bisoprolol	Worsened lipid profile
Metoprolol	Poor recovery from hypoglycaemia
	Sexual dysfunction
	Worsen claudication symptoms
Thiazide diuretics	
Bendrofluazide	Impairment of glucose tolerance
Chlorthalidone	Worsened lipid profile
Hydrochlorothiazide	Sexual dysfunction
etc.	Hypokalaemia
	May precipitate hyperosmolar state
Indapamide and frusemide have fewer problems	

When one agent alone (in full dosage) is insufficient, a second should be added; the same principles apply to the choice though most combinations are effective. ACE inhibitors should generally be combined with loop diuretics in increasing doses.

Lipids in diabetes

The level of plasma cholesterol is directly linked to death from macrovascular disease in the population as a whole. The same relationship is found in the diabetic.

Evidence from intervention and angiographic studies in the non-diabetic strongly suggests that the relationship is causative and that a 10% fall in plasma cholesterol is associated with a 20% fall in mortality. There is some evidence of atherosclerotic plaque regression with successful treatment. Consensus recommendations have now been made for lipid and lipoprotein levels in the general population and there is no reason to alter these for diabetes (Table 16.6).

Table 16.6 European recommendations for plasma lipid and lipoprotein levels

Lipid or lipoprotein	Recommended level
Total cholesterol	Less than 5.2 mmol/l
Triglyceride	Less than 2.3 mmol/l
HDL-cholesterol	Above 0.9 mmol/l

Lipids and diabetic control

Poorly-controlled patients with IDD or NIDD tend to have significantly raised LDL-cholesterol levels, which fall to normal with good control in IDD but not in NIDD. The protective HDL-cholesterol also tends to be normal, or even high, in IDD while it remains low in patients with NIDD even after control of hyperglycaemia. The exception in IDD is in patients with nephropathy, who have a high risk pattern of lipids (Table 16.7).

Patients may also have lipid disorders independent of their diabetes and a full family history is valuable.

Table 16.7 Summary of plasma lipid and lipoprotein changes in diabetes

Lipid or lipoprotein	Well-controlled IDD	IDD with nephropathy	Well-controlled NIDD
Total cholesterol	Normal	Increased	Increased
LDL cholesterol	Normal	Increased	Increased
HDL cholesterol	Normal/high	Decreased	Decreased
Triglyceride	Normal	Normal	Increased

Investigation

Except in special circumstances (e.g. eruptive xanthomata) measurement of lipids is not appropriate until acceptable control of diabetes has been achieved. While fasting triglyceride measurements are preferable, they are not always practicable and random determinations are adequate for screening though they may have to be repeated. Cholesterol is relatively little affected by eating.

When the hyperlipidaemia is confirmed other causes may need to be excluded (Table 16.8).

Treatment of hyperlipidaemia

Weight loss and diet are the two cornerstones of treatment and must be employed before drug therapy is commenced. Weight loss reduces LDL-cholesterol directly.

Table 16.8 Main causes of hyperlipidaemia other than diabetes

---

Primary hyperlipidaemias
Polygenic hypercholesterolaemia
Familial hypercholesterolaemia
Familial combined hyperlipidaemia
Familial hypertriglyceridaemia

Secondary causes
Renal impairment (including nephropathy)
Primary hypothyroidism
Alcohol excess
Thiazide diuretics
Beta-blockers

The dietary principles are simple and should aim at reduction of total fat intake to 30% or below of total calories with an increase in mono- and polyunsaturated fats and a reduction in saturated fat.

For IDD patients the best achievable control should be obtained and 3 months allowed to elapse on the diet before further measures are taken. In NIDD fewer patients will reach acceptable weight or glycaemic control targets but again an adequate time must be allowed before further measures are contemplated. Most authorities now advise that measures similar to those for the non-diabetic should be employed (Table 16.9).

Table 16.9 Graded management for hyperlipidaemia (mmol/l)

Cholesterol 5.0–6.5	Assess overall CVS risk factors Continue diet, weight loss Advise non-smoking Rarely medication
Cholesterol 6.5–7.8	Initially as for 5.0–6.5 Formal lipid-lowering diet + weight loss Monitor and consider adding drug therapy, especially if young and at high CVS risk
Cholesterol > 7.8	Full investigation for secondary causes Formal lipid-lowering diet + weight loss Appropriate drug therapy if level persists
Triglycerides 2.3–5.6	Identify and treat underlying causes Energy restriction and TG-lowering diet Exceptionally, appropriate drugs
Triglycerides > 5.6	As above, but drug therapy often required especially if pancreatitis has occurred.
Combined (cholesterol > 5.6 and triglycerides > 2.3)	Consider remnant hyperlipoproteinaemia or familial combined hyperlipidaemia Initially diet, with drugs if no response

Drug therapy for hyperlipidaemias

The indications for specific drug therapies remain unclear. There are two main groups of drugs (Table 16.10). The first cause a decrease in LDL-cholesterol particularly, and include the bile acid sequestrants, cholestyramine and colestipol, together with probucol. The major agent is cholestyramine which has however significant gastrointestinal side-effects.

The second group have wider effects, reducing triglycerides as well as LDL-cholesterol while increasing HDL-cholesterol. These include gemfibrozil and bezafibrate. Maxepa, the fish-oil derivate, is not yet adequately investigated.

New HMG-Co-reductase inhibitors such as simvastatin (already introduced) and lovastatin (expected shortly) appear to be much better tolerated and are effective lipid-lowering agents in diabetes, but experience is limited. In the UK simvastatin is being marketed for patients with cholesterol levels above 7.8 mmol/l.

Table 16.10 Use of lipid-lowering agents

Agent	Dose range	Special points
Cholestyramine	12–32 g/day	Needs fat-soluble vitamin supplements
Colestipol	5–30 g/day	Needs fat-soluble vitamin supplements
Probucol	1000 mg/day	Contraindicated in or just before pregnancy
Acipimox (nicotinic acid derivative)	500–750 mg/day	Contraindicated in pregnancy/lactation
Bezafibrate	400–600 mg/day	Avoid in severe renal or hepatic failure
Gemfibrozil	1200–1500 mg/day	Eyes and liver function need monitoring
Simvastatin	10–40 mg/day	Avoid in liver disease. Watch eyes and liver function

All these drugs have significant contraindications, requirements for monitoring or needs for supplements and significant side-effects. Recent copies of the *British National Formulary* and/or *MIMS* should be consulted before their prescription.

Smoking

Smoking is a major risk factor in diabetes as it is in the general population. No opportunity should be wasted to persuade patients to give up or, at the very least, to reduce their cigarette consumption.

Further reading

Jarrett R.J. (ed) (1984). *Diabetes and Heart Disease.* Elsevier, Amsterdam

Lewis B. (1988). Management of the hyperlipidaemic patient, *Journal of the Royal College of Physicians*; **22**, 28–31

Mogensen C.E. (ed) (1988). *The Kidney and Hypertension in Diabetes Mellitus.* Martinus Nijhoff, Boston

Taylor K.G. (ed) (1987). *Diabetes and the Heart.* Castle House Publications, Tunbridge Wells

17: The Diabetic Foot

The foot disorders of diabetes are common, distressing and may be debilitating. Considerable advances have recently been made in understanding the cause and improving the outlook for these patients.

Clinical features

The chief factors responsible for foot problems in diabetes are neuropathy and ischaemia or both together; the ischaemic foot is the more serious and the outlook less optimistic. The needs of investigation and treatment of these two groups of patients are so fundamentally different that they are divided into separate groups for their treatment in practice and for consideration in this chapter. Neuropathy results in a warm, numb, dry and normally painless foot in which pulses are palpable (Table 17.1); it leads to ulceration, Charcot joints and oedema. In contrast, the ischaemic foot is cold and pulses are absent; it is complicated by pain, ulceration from localized pressure, necrosis and gangrene. Foot deformities predispose to problems from ulceration, and sepsis plays havoc with both neuropathic and ischaemic feet.

Pathophysiology

THE NEUROPATHIC FOOT

Peripheral neuropathy leads to somatic sensory and autonomic damage (see Chapter 15). Small fibre damage predominates initially, causing loss of pain and temperature sensation and later a numb or even anaesthetic foot with loss of all sensory modalities. Sensory loss persists and abnormal forces which deform the foot occur unnoticed by the patient. Motor weakness is not commonly a feature of diabetic neuropathy although it probably causes weakness of the intrinsic foot muscles and leads to clawing of the toes.

Sympathetic damage causes loss of sweating and denervates peripheral blood vessels with profound effects. Absence of sweating results in a dry foot sometimes associated with cracked skin which acts as a portal of entry

Table 17.1 Characteristics of neuropathic and ischaemic foot ulcers

	Neuropathic	Ischaemic
Temperature	Warm	Cool
Pulses	Present	Absent
Pain	None	Severe
Site	Under toes and metatarsal heads	Lateral borders of feet

for sepsis. Vasomotor denervation causes a huge increase in peripheral blood flow, opening of arteriovenous shunts, and arterial medial degeneration with calcification. A warm foot associated with a very high blood flow (Fig. 17.1) which may be more than five times normal are characteristic features of the neuropathic foot. These major haemodynamic changes are at least in part responsible for oedema in the neuropathic foot which is a common finding, occasionally of considerable severity. Increase in bone blood flow also occurs (Fig. 17.2) and may cause osteopenia, and this could underly the development of the destructive bony changes of Charcot joints (Table 17.2).

Sympathetic denervation of the arteries to the foot also leads to increased vascular rigidity and medial calcification (Fig. 17.3) which is also commoner after lumbar sympathectomy. While there is no evidence that reduced blood flow results from this, Doppler examination of the foot circulation may give misleading results because of the incompressibility of the arteries (see p. 182).

Table 17.2 Circulatory changes in the neuropathic foot

Abnormality	Consequence
Increased foot circulation ⎱ Arteriovenous shunting ⎰	Oedema
Increased bone circulation	Osteopenia Charcot joints
Medial calcification	Rigid arteries; high brachial/ ankle systolic ratio (pressure index)

THE ISCHAEMIC LIMB

The blood supply to the foot is reduced by atherosclerosis of large vessels; the disease is commoner than in non-diabetics, but the histopathology is the same and only the distribution may be different. It is age-related and older patients and those who smoke are more likely to suffer foot problems from ischaemia.

Atheromatous plaques are usually extensive, bilateral and multi-segmental; in diabetics they are more likely to involve the distal vessels below the knee, so that tibial and peroneal obliteration are quite common. So-called 'small vessel' disease of arterioles and capillaries is a questionable entity and it is not known whether endothelial proliferation or basement membrane thickening have any significant effect on ischaemic lesions; their theoretical presence should in no way influence proper investigation and treatment of the ischaemic limb

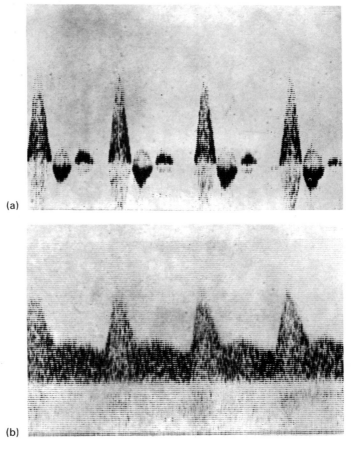

(a)

(b)

Fig. 17.1 Doppler sonagrams from the dorsalis pedis arteries of (a) a normal foot, and (b) a neuropathic foot. In the normal artery, forward flow occurs during systolic followed by reversed and then forward flow during diastole. The patterns in neuropathy slows the large diastolic flow with loss of reversal, indicating high arteriovenous shunting.

Precipitating causes of foot lesions

Foot damage and ulceration in both neuropathic and ischaemic feet always result from some noxious stimulus; in the neuropathic foot this may be unperceived by the patient and lesions may progress to an advanced stage before they are detected.

MECHANICAL INJURIES

The repetitive mechanical forces of normal gait often result in callus formation, especially in neuropathic patients. Callus develops at sites of

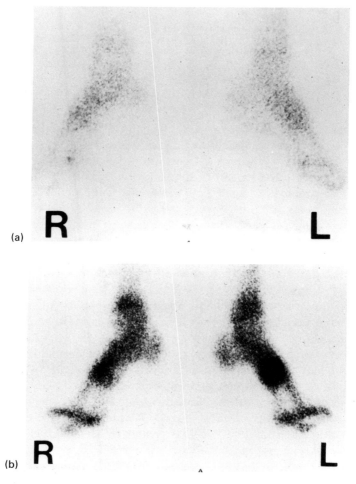

(a) R   L

(b) R   L

Fig. 17.2 Technetium diphosphonate isotope bone scans in (a) a normal foot, and (b) a neuropathic foot. The huge increase in uptake in the neuropathic foot represents the high bone blood flow. Radiographs were normal.

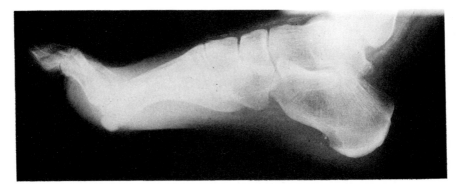

Fig. 17.3 Radiograph of a neuropathic foot showing marked arterial medial calcification. It also shows the effect of clawed toes causing protuberance of the metatarsal heads.

high pressure and therefore at various points of foot deformity as well as under the metatarsal heads. Tissue necrosis occurs deep to the plaque and eventually breaks to the surface with ulcer formation. The importance of pressure in the development of these lesions has been demonstrated by direct measurement of forces under the foot using pedobarography and vulnerable areas are those where pressure exceeds 10 kg/cm^2. Callus removal and alteration of points of high pressure by appropriate footwear are of the greatest important in both treatment and prevention.

Pressure from tight, ill-fitting shoes is a common cause of foot injury, blistering and subsequent sepsis. Shoes which do not accommodate deformities cause a particular hazard and new shoes, which should always be broken in gradually, are frequently the culprits. Oedema poses special problems especially if it varies a great deal and this needs special consideration.

Direct mechanical injuries are common. They occur mainly from stones or protuberant nails inside shoes, or when patients with insensitive feet walk barefoot and encounter sharp objects.

Burns cause blistering with subsequent infection. Hot water bottle burns are the most frequent cause, but unpleasant lesions occur in some neuropathic patients who may fall asleep with their feet too close to an open fire or actually resting on a radiator. Bathing in excessively hot water, or walking barefoot on hot sand during seaside holidays may also cause serious burns.

Chemical injuries occur from the use of keratolytic agents, notably 'corn plasters'; these contain a high concentraton of salicylic acid and may cause liquefaction of tissues, sepsis and necrosis which may lead to surgery and amputation. They should never be used by diabetics.

SEPSIS

Infection gains entry following abrasion of the skin resulting from any of the traumas described above, or just through cracks in hard, dry skin which may develop spontaneously. Sometimes interdigital fungal infection (athlete's foot) serves as the portal of entry. Sepsis is the major cause of the evolution of foot lesions converting simple ulcers into horrendous foot disease.

The organisms are usually *Staphylococcus aureus* or streptococci; anaerobes flourish when there is a deep infection and include bacteroides and more rarely clostridium perfringens.

Lesions

NEUROPATHIC LESIONS

The neuropathic ulcer develops typically at points of high pressure in relation to areas of heavy callus formation (Fig. 17.4; Table 17.3). They most often occur under the tips of the toes, under the metatarsal heads, concealed as interdigital ulcers and occasionally on the heel. Less frequently they are seen on the dorsum of the toes and over bunions. They are frequently circular, punched out in appearance and painless.

Following the entry of sepsis the picture changes, sometimes rapidly. Cellulitis spreads fast, and deep involvement of the foot with abscess formation causes the foot to become dusky red, swollen and even painful; the development of pain usually indicates the need for urgent surgery. Local arterial thrombosis causes digital gangrene. Subcutaneous gas formation can occasionally be felt on palpation and seen on radiographs.

The development of osteomyelitis (Fig. 17.5) is always serious because it

Table 17.3 Sites of ulceration in neuropathic and ischaemic feet

Site	Neuropathic	Ischaemic
Toes	68%	59%
Metatarsal		
Plantar	20%	3%
Lateral	3%	18%
Other	9%	20%

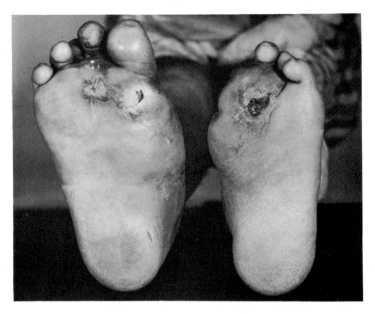

Fig. 17.4 Neuropathic ulcers. The surrounding callus, symmetry of the lesions, clawing of the toes and digital amputations are all characteristic.

can rarely be eradicated without surgical excision. Sometimes fragments of dead bone are extruded through open wounds.

In conclusion, neuropathic ulceration and subsequent sepsis develop in a warm, insensitive foot with bounding pulses. There is no pain unless deep sepsis and abscess formation occur.

Neuroarthropathy of the Charcot joint (Figs 17.6 and 17.7) is a rare complication which develops in a few neuropathic diabetics. Severe bone and joint destruction occurs most frequently in the metatarsal–tarsal region and less commonly at the metatarsophalangeal, ankle or sub-talar joints.

The initial presentation is with a hot, swollen and erythematous foot, which aches in one-third of cases; it is frequently misdiagnosed as cellulitis or gout. The precipitating cause is commonly minor trauma such as tripping or a mild sprain which may even be ignored at the time. At this early stage plain X-rays are normal, though isotope bone scans are grossly abnormal showing considerably increased isotope uptake. During the following weeks rapid bony destruction and joint dislocations occur, with grotesque appearance of new bone formation at sites of damage. The foot deforms and classically develops both a rocker bottom deformity because of downward displacement of the tarsus, and medial convexity resulting from displacement of the talonavicular joint or tarso-metatarsal dislocation. The

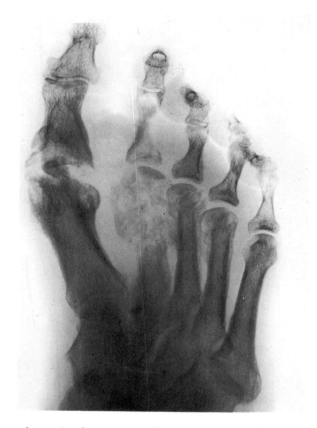

Fig. 17.5 Bony destruction from osteomyelitis in a neuropathic foot.

evolution of these changes occurs over 2–3 months after which the foot seems to stabilize. Friction within ill fitting shoes may further aggravate these problems by causing new areas of ulceration.

Treatment aims to alleviate early symptoms and attempts to prevent the appearance of major deformity, although there is no certainty that this can be done. During the acute stage bed rest is important and the use of drugs such as indomethacin can reduce the intensity of the inflammatory response. Non-weight-bearing is advisable for some weeks, either by the use of crutches or non-walking plaster cast. When deformities develop it is essential to provide individually made shoes to prevent further friction and ulceration.

Neuropathic oedema is common in the neuropathic foot and causes problems from friction inside shoes which cannot accommodate the swollen foot; it results from the major haemodynamic changes already described, and is occasionally severe and intractable.

Treatment of neuropathic oedema can be by conventional diuretic treatment, but the use of the sympathomimetic agent ephedrine is specific and effective. Initially, ephedrine 30 mg tds is used and can be increased to 60 mg tds. Side effects and tachyphylaxis do not seem to arise.

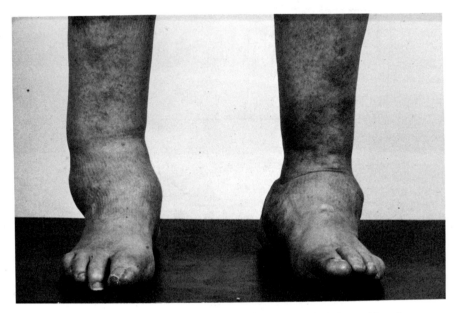

Fig. 17.6 Charcot (neuroarthropathic) joints. The feet are grossly deformed from bony destruction and dislocation; the 'rocker' sole is characteristic.

ISCHAEMIC LESIONS

The commonest manifestation is painful ulceration presenting as areas of superficial necrosis, surrounded by a rim of erythema. The lesions occur chiefly on the great toe or the lateral borders of the feet overlying the 1st and 5th metatarsal heads. The ulcers are shallow, not associated with callus and quite distinct from those occurring in the neuropathic foot; foot pulses are, of course, absent (Table 17.3).

The development of rest pain in the pink, ischaemic foot is always ominous. Digital gangrene may follow, and spread, and is a much more serious event than in the neuropathic foot with its good circulation. These changes in the ischaemic foot nearly always require major amputation.

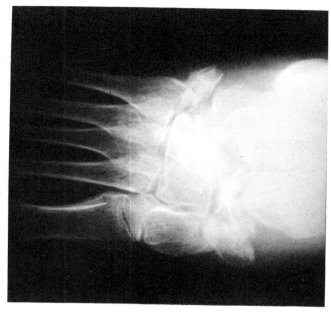

Fig. 17.7 Charcot (neuroarthropathic) joints: radiographs showing dislocation of the mid-tarsal joint, bone destruction and new bone formation.

The introduction of sepsis into the ischaemic foot adds to the severity of the situation and demands urgent attention.

Claudication in a diabetic with ischaemia requires the same attention as in others. It may persist for years without causing serious problems, and in some instances it disappears spontaneously. Claudication alone infrequently requires surgical intervention, although with the development of new and simpler techniques such as angioplasty, this situation may change.

Investigation

Inspection

The foot is inspected for deformities, notably clawing of the toes, pes cavus, hallux rigidus, bunions or the more severe abnormalities of Charcot foot changes. Examination of footwear is highly relevant.

Assessment of neuropathy

Clinical assessment should be undertaken, including knee and ankle reflexes and simple sensory tests, although these may fail to detect pain and temperature sensory deficits. The use of a Biothesiometer is of value to measure vibration perception threshold; a reading of more than 35 volts indicates feet at risk of ulceration.

Microbiological cultures

Swabs should always be taken from the base of an ulcer, or after débridement of deeper lesions. Blood cultures are taken when cellulitis, fever and systemic illness is present.

Circulation

Palpation of foot pulses is mandatory; if one or both are present, the prognosis is usually good and vascular investigations are not necessary. If they are both absent, proximal pulses should also be assessed, and proper vascular investigations performed as follows:

DOPPLER ASSESSMENT AND MEASUREMENT OF THE PRESSURE INDEX

The pressure index is the ratio of the ankle systolic to brachial systolic pressure. Simple Doppler equipment is cheap and of great value in the foot clinic. The pressure index is normally 1.0–1.2: a ratio less than 0.9 indicates ischaemia and, when it is less than 0.6, severe ischaemia is present and the prognosis poor. False elevation of this index is unfortunately common because of rigidity and calcification of vessels so that high readings may be spurious.

ANGIOGRAPHY

Angiography is needed if ischaemic foot ulcers do not resolve in 1 month, or if more serious lesions such as rest pain with or without gangrene develops.

Foot pressures

Simple foot pressure pads yield some information regarding sites of excessive pressure. More sophisticated pedobarography should in future identify these areas and also assist in determining appropriate footwear needed to alleviate these high pressure areas.

Management

General measures for neuropathic and ischaemic feet

These comprise four distinct aspects:

CHIROPODY

This is needed to remove callus and permit efficient drainage in the neuropathic foot, and for wound débridement from both neuropathic and ischaemic lesions. Simple ulcers are treated with antiseptic applications (savlidil) and non-adhesive dry dressings.

ERADICATION OF INFECTION

This is urgent if cellulitis develops, and after admission to hospital. Intravenous benzyl penicillin and flucloxacillin are used because *Staphylococcus aureus* and streptococci are the commonest organisms; usually metronidazole is added as well especially with deep-seated necrotic lesions. For less acute situations, oral antibiotics are used. Where penicillin allergy is a problem, erythromycin is given instead. When cultures clearly reveal a different pattern of infection, appropriate antibiotics are given. Our usual practice is to continue antibiotics until the lesion has healed because of the high relapse rate when they are stopped, even though clear proof of the effectiveness of this policy has not been obtained from controlled trials.

Local treatment of infected lesions is by saline irrigation two or three times daily.

REDUCTION OF WEIGHT-BEARING FORCES

In the acute stages bed rest with the limb elevated is important and both heels must be protected from blistering by elevation on a simple foam wedge (Figs 17.8 & 17.9); otherwise non-weight-bearing is achieved by the use of crutches or total-contact walking plaster. In the longer term, specially fitted shoes are needed to ensure redistribution of weight-bearing forces and alleviation of pressure at vulnerable sites. Further details on shoes are presented on p. 189. The total-contact plaster cast is of great value and permits walking while removing pressure from the lesion. The cast is effective because it greatly increases the surface area of contact. The important difference from a conventional below-knee plaster is the innermost layer of plaster (which is a thin shell applied loosely), and modelled to conform easily to the foot and leg.

SURGICAL INTERVENTION

Surgery is needed to drain pus and to excise necrotic tissue, and when possible in cases of ischaemia, to improve the circulation by angioplasty or arterial surgery.

In the neuropathic foot with an intact circulation, swelling, inflammation and pain indicate the development of an abscess needing urgent surgical

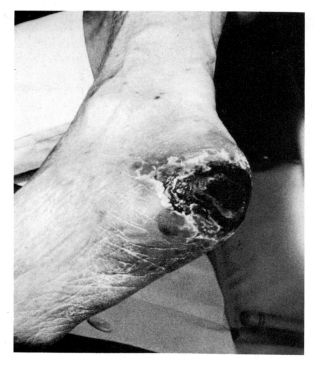

Fig. 17.8 Heel ulcer in an ischaemic foot which developed following a laparotomy because of inadequate heel protection. Below-knee amputation followed.

drainage. Digital gangrene obviously requires local amputation although the presence of extensive sepsis in the foot in such cases demands the more extensive resection of a ray amputation in which the digit and distal metatarsal are removed; this operation is usually highly successful and rapid healing is expected. The presence of osteomyelitis is usually an indication for surgery since infection tends to relapse repeatedly in these patients. Radical amputations are rarely needed in neuropathic limbs with a good circulation, and when they are required, it is usually because the patient has come for advice too late.

Surgery for the ischaemic foot is described below.

Management of the ischaemic foot

The problems in the ischaemic foot are those of ulceration, gangrene, sepsis and pain. If extensive gangrene is present, major amputation (usually

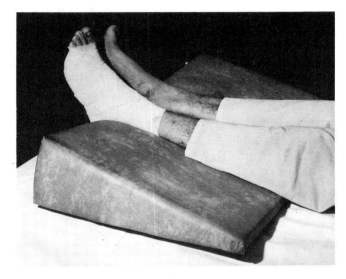

Fig. 17.9 Foam wedge used to protect the heels of all diabetics requiring bed rest.

below-knee) should be performed as soon as possible. When digital gangrene occurs decisions regarding treatment are never easy since digital or ray amputations rarely if ever succeed and should not normally be attempted. Limited operations in the ischaemic foot (other than wound débridement or drainage of pus) have earned the diabetic foot its bad reputation and may lead to many months of fruitless hospital treatment.

The following plan of investigation and treatment is adopted:

MEDICAL MANAGEMENT

Rest, antibiotics, chiropody and elimination of oedema are always needed, and have been described in detail on p. 183. Drainage of pus or wound débridement may also be required. More than 70% of ischaemic ulcers are expected to heal using simple conservative measures.

Where limited dry digital gangrene is present, when sepsis has been eradicated and arterial reconstruction is not feasible, it is best not to amputate the digit but to continue conservative treatment with regular attendance for review and continuing chiropody until the necrotic digit auto-amputates itself. Attempts at surgical amputation usually fail because they do not heal and ultimately result in below-knee amputation. This conservative approach saves many patients from suffering major amputations (Fig. 17.10).

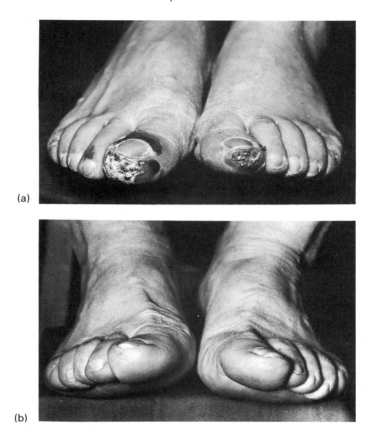

(a)

(b)

Fig. 17.10 Terminal gangrene of the great toes (a) and recovery with conservative treatment (b).

SURGICAL MANAGEMENT

Arterial reconstruction, angioplasty and amputation are the surgical options available for treating the ischaemic foot.

The chief indications for attempting arterial reconstruction or angioplasty are intractable rest pain especially in the pink, painful ischaemic foot, and ulceration that has not responded to medical treatment. When limited gangrene develops the need for major amputation is just occasionally averted by surgical improvement of the blood supply.

Diabetes is not itself a contraindication to vascular surgery or angioplasty. It is the nature and site of the lesions which determine the procedure to be adopted. Aorto-iliac, aortofemoral or femoropopliteal bypass operations are performed as appropriate; in the future, microvascular surgery may enable more distal arterial lesions to be tackled by vascular surgeons performing femorotibial bypass operations.

Balloon angioplasty in which intraluminal balloons are used to dilate stenoses in obstructed arteries (Fig. 17.11) is a major advance and can be used in patients too frail for major vascular surgery. Lesions which can be treated by angioplasty should be less than 10 cm in length. Iliac artery angioplasties are the most successful and those below the trifurcation of the popliteal artery least so. We now have some evidence that intractable ischaemic ulcers will heal more quickly after successful angioplasty.

As with vascular surgery, the most distal arterial occlusions remain difficult to treat; laser angioplasty still needs to be investigated.

AMPUTATION

The need for below-knee amputations should not necessarily be considered as a failure of treatment — appropriately-timed surgery and rehabilitation are often more successful than prolonged and fruitless attempts at

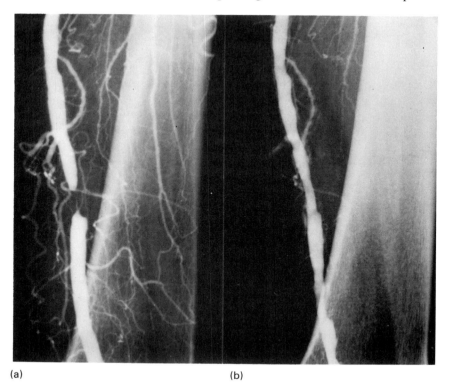

(a)   (b)

Fig. 17.11 Atheromatous narrowing of the superficial femoral artery before (a) and after (b) balloon angioplasty.

conservative treatment. Surgical sympathectomy is rarely performed now, and its usefulness in alleviating ischaemic pain very limited; it can be tried when other measures have failed but it does not significantly improve blood flow.

Indications for below-knee amputation include extensive gangrene, or more limited gangrene in the presence of gross sepsis. Intractable pain which cannot be relieved by other measures is occasionally an indication for amputation even if the lesions themselves are relatively minor. Limited operations including digital or ray amputations rarely, if ever, succeed in the ischaemic foot unless the blood supply can be improved surgically; the choice then lies between the more radical below knee amputation or conservative treatment leading to auto-amputation (see p. 185). Major amputations can be performed readily and rapidly even in very sick, elderly patients. There is often a spectacular improvement in the general condition and well-being of patients especially when sepsis has been present, and these operations should not be delayed. Fortunately above-knee amputations are rarely needed.

Prevention

Prevention of foot ulcers and sepsis, and in particular preventing their recurrence is an exceptionally important aspect of diabetic care; of all the complications of diabetes, the foot problems can be the most successfully averted.

KING'S COLLEGE HOSPITAL – DIABETIC DEPARTMENT

CARE OF YOUR FEET

To help prevent complications:–

DO
wash daily with soap and water.
dry well, especially between toes.
change socks/stockings daily.
see that your shoes are not too tight.
see a Chiropodist.

DON'T
walk barefoot.
sit too close to a fire or radiator.
put your feet on hot water bottles.
neglect even slight injuries – see your Doctor.
attempt your own chiropody – see your Chiropodist.

KCH 247

Fig. 17.12 Example of simple printed instructions regarding footcare.

1   Education. Every diabetic needs to be made aware of the potential hazards to the feet and the methods by which they can be avoided. This is done first at diagnosis, but the advice needs to be reinforced at intervals and is most easily done at chiropody attendances. All patients should receive simple printed instructions regarding footcare, an example of which is shown in Fig 17.12.

2   Chiropody. Neuropathic ulcers often begin deep to callus (see p. 177). Regular attention by a chiropodist is the single most important measure needed to prevent foot ulceration. Furthermore, the spread of sepsis can also be prevented if emergency facilities are available so that patients can be seen and treated at the earliest sign of a lesion. Relief of pressure points either by specially fitted shoes or insoles can also be provided by chiropodists. A proper chiropody service is now an essential part of diabetic care which should not be neglected.

3   Foot inspection. This is routinely undertaken at diagnosis and regular intervals when the diabetes and its complications are brought under review. Structural deformities are sought, and examination for the presence of vascular disease and neuropathy is important.

4   Shoes and insoles. Correctly-fitting shoes are vital in ulcer prevention. They must accommodate any deformities and reduce pressure at major pressure points to eliminate recurring callus formation. Sometimes shoes must be specially made for an individual patient, which is, of course, expensive; there is however an increasing range of standard shoes providing sufficient depth to accommodate appropriate insoles. Sometimes provision of insoles alone will suffice. While chiropodists can provide a part of the shoe-fitting service, and often themselves make the insoles, attendance at the foot clinic by an orthotist or shoe fitter is also extremely important, so that patients can be measured and fitted with proper shoes on the spot.

Conclusions

It is now possible both to prevent diabetic foot problems and to treat them successfully. More than 90% of neuropathic ulcers and 70% of ischaemic ulcers are expected to heal. The organization of diabetic foot care is extremely important and one of the most optimistic aspects of diabetic management.

Further reading

Connor H., Boulton A.J.M. & Ward J.D. (eds) (1987). *The Foot in Diabetes*. John Wiley & Sons, Chichester
Levin M.E. & O'Neal W. (eds) (1988). *The Diabetic Foot*, 3rd edn. Mosby, St Louis

Section 4
Special Situations

18: Diabetes, Pregnancy and Contraception

The successful outcome of most diabetic pregnancies represents one of the major achievements of modern medicine. Perinatal mortality among offspring of IDD mothers at King's has fallen from approximately 30% in the 1940s to about 2% in the last 10 years (Fig. 18.1). This represents not only advances in diabetic care but the result of very close liaison with obstetric and neonatal paediatric colleagues.

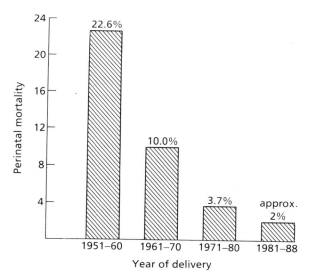

Fig. 18.1 Perinatal mortality to mothers with IDD from 1951–1988 at King's College Hospital.

Pregnancy

There are two clearly defined situations to be considered: (1) pregnancy in an established insulin-dependent diabetic; and (2) non-insulin-dependent diabetes or impaired glucose tolerance presenting in pregnancy.

193

While IDD can present in pregnancy and established NIDD may occur before pregnancy, both are very uncommon problems in Caucasian populations.

Control of carbohydrate metabolism in pregnancy

The normal woman shows some deterioration of glucose tolerance in pregnancy, mainly in the last trimester. This appears to be related to the physiological and hormonal changes of pregnancy, inducing insulin resistance and requiring increased secretion or provision of insulin. There is also a fall in the renal threshold for glucose. As a result of this insulin resistance, insulin requirements of the established diabetic increase substantially during pregnancy.

Gestational diabetes

Those women who develop diabetes in pregnancy are described as gestational diabetics, and the usual WHO criteria for glucose tolerance are used. Reclassification is necessary after delivery. Some of them will then remain diabetic while most will revert to normal glucose tolerance; the test is normally performed 6 weeks after delivery. As many as half of those who have had gestational diabetes will become diabetic in later life.

Those patients with impaired glucose tolerance (IGT) in pregnancy are usually treated as if they were diabetic. There is however conflicting evidence as to whether this abnormality is associated with much, if any, increased risk to the foetus. The recommendations of the National Diabetes Data Group (NDDG) in the USA for interpretation of glucose tolerance in pregnancy differ from those of the WHO, but this controversy does not have significant practical implications.

Oral hypoglycaemic agents are rarely used in diabetic pregnancy. There is no clear evidence of foetal toxicity but most physicians avoid them, preferring the optimal control obtainable with insulin and regarding any potential risk as unacceptable.

Physiology of maternal hyperglycaemia and its effect on the foetus

Glucose freely crosses the placenta and thus maternal hyperglycaemia is reflected in the foetal circulation. Foetal metabolism is thus much more dependent upon the flux of metabolites across the placental barrier. Insulin however does not cross the placenta and glucoregulation in the foetus is thus dependent on foetal insulin production. Differentiated B-cells have been noted in the foetus as early as 11 days, but there is dispute as to when normal secretory function begins; the normal foetal islet appears less responsive than the adult one to glucose though fully responsive to amino acids. Direct measurement however suggests that even mild 'passive' hyperglycaemia leads to hyperinsulinism in the foetus. The foetal pancreas is hyperfunctional late in pregnancy, and at birth when the maternal connection is severed this can cause hypoglycaemia in the foetus until it readjusts. On the other hand there is no good evidence that maternal hypoglycaemia is harmful to the foetus. Furthermore, excess insulin does not cross the placenta and the foetal liver is already producing glucose from an early stage of pregnancy. However maternal hypoglycaemia is common in the first trimester especially and often requires rapid adjustments to insulin therapy.

Pregnancy in the established insulin-dependent diabetic

Fertility appears to be normal among diabetic women, although some choose not to have children because of the small risk of their becoming diabetic or because they already have major complications. There is a slightly increased risk of abortion for poorly-controlled patients only.

The main problems associated with diabetic pregnancy are:

AN INCREASED INCIDENCE OF CONGENITAL ABNORMALITIES

This appears to be mainly due to glycaemic control in the critical early weeks of pregnancy (2–6) when organogenesis is taking place. Most studies suggest that poor control at this time (an HbA1 more than 50% above the upper limit of normal) is associated with a 2–4-fold increase in abnormality rate. Congenital abnormalities are decreased amongst diabetics who are able to achieve good control peri-conceptually and therefore during the very earliest weeks of pregnancy.

The overall UK abnormality rate in 1979–80 was 4.3%. The abnormalities are those occurring in the general population: they include skeletal abnormalities such as spina bifida or hemivertebra, congenital heart disease and neurological defects such as microcephaly or anencephaly. Sacral agenesis is greatly increased in diabetes but is still extremely uncommon.

LATE INTRA-UTERINE DEATH

Unexplained intra-uterine deaths in the third trimester are very uncommon, but still may occur more frequently than in the general population. Previously they were so frequent that diabetic infants were routinely delivered several weeks early to avoid this problem, but this practice resulted in neonatal deaths from respiratory distress syndrome, now virtually eliminated. When intra-uterine deaths do occur there is often no apparent warning, even from such modern techniques as 'kick charts' or foetal heart rate monitoring. Recent evidence suggests that they may be due to foetal hypoxia although the primary cause of this, apart from a general statement of placental insufficiency, is not clear.

TIMING OF DELIVERY

This is very important. We now allow diabetic pregnancies to proceed to full term unless there are obstetric reasons for early delivery.

There has been considerable controversy about the optimum time for delivery of infants of diabetic mothers. Until about 10 years ago, delivery usually took place around 36 weeks, this being judged to be the time where the risks of prematurity (especially respiratory distress syndrome) became less than the risk of intra-uterine death if the pregnancy was allowed to continue. The incidence of intra-uterine death has fallen dramatically and many centres now allow otherwise uncomplicated patients to go to term and enter spontaneous labour, thus reducing the Caesarian section rate. Others are more conservative and would recommend induction of labour at about 38–39 weeks. The incidence of failed inductions leads to a higher rate of Caesarian sections, but both policies are associated with very good results in the best centres.

MACROSOMIA

The classical diabetic infant is large, fat and plethoric. This 'macrosomia' is usually defined as a baby above an absolute weight (e.g. 4 kg) or, more usefully, greater than the 95th centile for the gestational age. The cause is not clear, although it probably relates at least in part to the growth promoting activities of insulin or insulin-like growth factors, which are raised in the diabetic foetus even when glycaemic control is very good. Recent evidence suggests that the birth weight distribution of babies born to diabetic mothers is shifted by about 500 g above that of the non-diabetic population when corrected for gestational age. An example growth chart is shown in Fig. 18.2.

The problems relating to macrosomia are largely mechanical, namely the increased difficulty of delivery by the vaginal route leading to such problems as shoulder dystocia and thus to an increased instrumental and Caesarian section rate. There is also an increased chance of birth injury. These problems may increase with the trend to full-term delivery.

Macrosomia has not been greatly reduced by immaculate control of

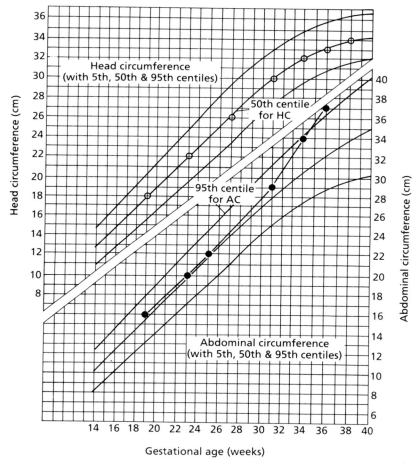

Fig. 18.2 Example of foetal growth chart showing abdominal circumference with development of macrosomia in the second trimester onwards.

diabetes during pregnancy but, even with this degree of control, mean blood glucose levels are still higher than normal.

NEONATAL HYPOGLYCAEMIA

The physiology of this problem has been discussed above. All babies of diabetic mothers require regular monitoring of blood glucose for 24 hours after delivery, ideally using BM sticks every 1–2 hours. Frequent feeding is often sufficient treatment, but glucose infusion may be necessary where the problem is severe or if the baby will not feed well.

Polycythaemia, hyperbilirubinaemia and hypocalcaemia are commoner among these infants.

Diabetic management during pregnancy

In previous years most patients were admitted for part, or even all, of pregnancy. This is no longer considered necessary and perinatal mortality has fallen despite the more liberal approach. It is however essential for the patient to be in contact with expert advice regularly and most would advise a minimum of fortnightly visits up to about week 32 or 36, and then weekly until delivery. Optimal results have been obtained in joint specialist clinics where both diabetic physicians and interested obstetricians manage the patients jointly; there is no place for non-specialists making occasional forays into this area. For intelligent and well-controlled patients, especially those with long distances to travel, occasional visits may be replaced by telephone consultations dealing with the purely diabetic problems.

The management of IDD in pregnancy is generally not difficult. The patients are almost always well motivated and the general principles of insulin treatment remain unchanged.

INSULIN REQUIREMENTS IN IDD

In the established IDD patient insulin requirements during pregnancy stay roughly static during the first trimester, and may fall slightly. Thereafter they rise progressively to a mean of about twice the pre-pregnant levels though this varies from a small increase (25–50%) up to a fourfold or greater increase. The peak is usually reached at about 32–36 weeks after which a slight fall may occur (Fig. 18.3).

Some particular points are as follows:

1 Hypoglycaemia. Though mean insulin requirements do not greatly alter in the first trimester, many patients develop quite marked hypoglycaemia. Whether this is related to decreased food intake from nausea is not clear, but rapid corrective action by reduction and adjustment of dose is vital as is frequent home monitoring. Occasionally patients need to be admitted at this stage as the problem may cause loss of confidence quite apart from the intrinsic dangers of hypoglycaemia itself.

2 Insulin regimes. The usual insulin regimes (Chapter 9) are applicable; any regime is satisfactory as long as it obtains good control without hypoglycaemia. For insulin-dependent patients twice daily mixed regimes of short and intermediate acting insulins are the minimum; many patients manage better with insulin three times daily using mixed insulins in the morning, short acting at supper time and an intermediate acting insulin at bedtime — this is particularly beneficial for those troubled by nocturnal

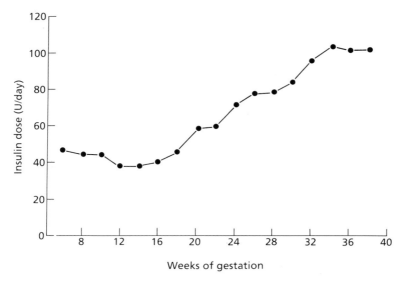

Fig. 18.3 Example of usual changes in insulin requirements in a patient with IDD.

hypoglycaemia. Multiple injection regimes, including use of the pens, are also valuable although they do not necessarily lead to better control than optimized conventional regimes. A very high standard of control is relatively easy to achieve during pregnancy.

3 Persistent poor control. This is another indication for short term admission as it usually indicates poor compliance with one or more aspects of treatment. It is more common in the very young, the single and those with a history of longstanding poor control. Full re-evaluation of all aspects of treatment including diet and injection techniques and sites, and monitoring, should be undertaken.

4 Targets for control. In most patients, if there are no exceptional circumstances, the aim should be to obtain pre-prandial glucose readings of 3.5–6 mmol/l and post-prandial levels not exceeding 8 mmol/l. The target for HbA1 should be within the normal range, although it is difficult to reduce it below the upper part of the range without causing unacceptable hypoglycaemia.

MONITORING

Good quality home monitoring is important throughout pregnancy. In the early stages and when there are problems this may need to be up to 7 times daily, but in most patients less frequent readings (1–4 times daily) give sufficient information. An example is shown in Fig. 18.4. Meter readings are obviously preferable, but adequate results are obtained with visual readings

MONTH		TEST TIME							INSULIN A.M.		INSULIN P.M.		COMMENTS
Day	Date	Before B/Fast	After B/Fast	Before Lunch	After Lunch	Before Dinner	Evening	Before Bed	Clear	Cloudy	Clear	Cloudy	
	1												
	2												
	3												
	4												
	5												
	6												
	7												
	8												
	9												
	10												
	11												
	12												
	13												
	14												
	15												
	16												
	17												
	18												
	19								BRKFST	LUNCH	SUP	BED	
Sun	20	5.7	6.2	8.3	5.3	8.9	6.2	8.2	16	14	14	110	
Mon	21	7.7		6.1	5.8	7.7		8.7					
Tues	22	4.8					7.9						
Wed	23	3.8	6.7	10.2		46	9.2	6.0					
Thurs	24	5.9		7.6	5.2	5.3	5.6						
Fri	25	3.2	6.9	6.3	4.7	9.7		9.5					
Sat	26	3.4	6.7	8.8	6.7	6.0		5.5					
	27												
	28												
	29												
	30												
	31												

BLOOD GLUCOSE MMOL/l — 20, 15, 10, 5, 2, 0

DIET:

Fig. 18.4 Example of blood glucose monitoring in pregnancy.

especially if these are checked in the laboratory early in the pregnancy.

The use of glycosylated haemoglobin has proved very valuable although it takes some weeks to reflect changes in glycaemic control. We measure HbA1 at every clinic visit. Its greatest value is to confirm good or bad control when compared with the patient's own blood glucose readings and also to bring attention to those patients in whom there are discrepancies. The use of fructosamine as an alternative and more rapidly responsive index remains controversial and is not generally advised.

NEPHROPATHY

Pregnancy in established diabetic nephropathy is undesirable chiefly because of the mother's limited life expectancy. If however patients ignore advice, then a successful pregnancy is possible and does not alter the rate of development of diabetic renal disease. The foetal outcome is less predictable than in those with uncomplicated diabetes; hypertension is frequently a problem, foetal growth may be retarded and premature delivery of small babies is not uncommon. Successful pregnancies have been recorded in those with renal transplants.

RETINOPATHY

Diabetic retinopathy may worsen during pregnancy. Whether this is a specific effect of the pregnancy or due to the considerable and rapid improvements in control that accompany it is not known. Fundal examination at the begining of every pregnancy and at regular intervals is mandatory, especially in those with pre-existing retinopathy.

Management of gestational diabetes

The initial management of gestational diabetes is by diet. Those patients with marked hyperglycaemia, random glucose levels above 11–13 mmol/l, are not likely to be controlled adequately by diet alone and should be started immediately on insulin. In this situation twice daily intermediate or ready-mixed insulins are often satisfactory. This can be started as an outpatient, though education and training have to be undertaken without delay. Patients need to be taught home blood glucose monitoring and the aims of therapy should be the same as those for IDD (see above). Failure of diet alone as indicated by random blood glucose levels of more than 7 mmol/l or fasting levels of more than 5–6 mmol/l should lead to a transfer to insulin, although if this only occurs in the last 4–8 weeks of pregnancy it is probably of little benefit to the foetus.

Gestational diabetics are prone to macrosomia and late intra-uterine death in the same way as those with established IDD.

Obstetric problems

Diabetic patients, both IDD and gestational, are liable to any of the usual complications of pregnancy. Some of these, in particular (poly)hydramnios and pregnancy-induced hypertension (pre-eclampsia) may be more common among diabetics. These, as with all other obstetric complications, are managed in the same way as in the normal subject though the diabetic team should always remain closely involved to prevent inadvertent loss of control during anaesthesia or other stressful procedures.

Two particular situations require mention. The use of steroids, to induce lung maturation, or beta-sympathomimetic agents (salbutamol) to delay labour are both associated with immediate worsening of diabetic control which occurs within 1–2 hours. Our practice is to use an insulin pump or infusion in addition to continuation of the usual insulin regime for as long as proves necessary. This should be started immediately; a high infusion rate is sometimes needed varying from 2 to more than 12 U/hour (see p. 107).

Delivery

Vaginal delivery should be performed unless there are obstetric indications to the contrary. Caesarian section rates remain high however, and over 50% of our deliveries are still by this means. The indications for Caesarian section are: (1) normal obstetric indications for Caesarian section; (2) two or more previous Caesarian sections; (3) actual or presumed difficulty of delivery because of macrosomia.

DIABETIC MANAGEMENT DURING LABOUR

This should follow the guidelines for the management of any surgical procedure (see Chapter 11). An insulin pump should be used until the time of delivery; most patients need between 0.5 and 2 U/hour to maintain the blood glucose between 3 and 6 mmol/l. It should then be stopped immediately though glucose should continue to run for a few minutes longer to allow the insulin to clear. In the conscious patient, it is usually sufficient not to give any more insulin until the patient takes her first meal. It is then essential to reduce the insulin dose to the pre-pregnancy regime; if this is not done, catastrophic hypoglycaemia may occur. One to 2-hourly blood glucose readings should be taken after delivery to avoid loss of control.

Breast feeding

Diabetic mothers may breast feed normally. As an empirical rule the dietary carbohydrate should be increased by approximately 50 g daily and this is very conveniently taken as milk.

Questions women ask

Should I, as a diabetic, have a baby? Except in the rare instances of severe complications (see above) the answer is yes.

Will the baby be normal? If diabetic control is good before conception there is little if any increased risk of abnormalities. Even in those with poor control the overall risk is about double that of the normal population.

What is the chance of the baby becoming diabetic? If only the mother has IDD, about 1–2% by age 25.

Do hypos harm the baby? There is no evidence that this is the case, but they should be prevented for the mother's sake.

Screening for diabetes in pregnancy

Screening is needed to detect gestational diabetes. We now measure random blood glucose at 26–28 weeks gestation and use the following criteria to indicate the need for a glucose tolerance test:

Random blood glucose > 5.6 mmol/l more than 2 hours after a meal.
Random blood glucose > 6.1 mmol/l within 2 hours of a meal.
Previous history of glucose intolerance in pregnancy
Foetal macrosomia (abdominal circumference above 95th centile)

If glycosuria occurs, a random blood glucose estimation should be performed and interpreted as above. The rare cases of IDD presenting in pregnancy should be easy to diagnose.

Pre-pregnancy counselling

With the recognition that congenital abnormality rates are related to mean glycaemic control in the early weeks of pregnancy, it becomes essential to improve diabetic control before conception. As well as providing the opportunity to improve control by education, more intensive monitoring and, where appropriate, altering insulin regimes, these counselling clinics provide an ideal opportunity to deal with the anxieties and queries of the diabetic mothers. It is our policy to mark the notes of all women of child-bearing age and to ask regularly if a pregnancy is planned. If not, and if they are sexually active, then arrangements for contraception are discussed (see below).

In common with many other clinics the attendance rate before pregnancy is only about 40% and those who become pregnant without counselling are more frequently in the high risk groups, in particular the young, the unmarried and those with the worst control.

Contraception

A planned pregnancy is important for diabetic patients and contraception therefore assumes even greater significance than normal. Potentially deleterious effects of the sex hormones on carbohydrate and lipid tolerance are however probably more important in NIDD patients and those with impaired glucose intolerance rather than in IDD patients where insulin is already being administered exogenously. With the low-dose (20–30 mg of oestrogen) combined pills the biochemical changes are minimal and these are now considered acceptable for IDD patients except those with nephropathy, ischaemic heart disease, hypertension or hyperlipidaemia, in whom alternative methods of contraception should be used. The same applies for smokers, in whom the risks of oral contraception are greater. An alternative policy is the use of the progesterone-only pills, though these are less effective in contraceptive terms and frequently cause amenorrhoea.

The choice of alternative methods of contraception is essentially the same as in the non-diabetic patient. When the family is complete, male or female sterilization has much to commend it.

Further reading

Brudenell J.M. & Doddridge M. (1989). *Diabetic Pregnancy*. Churchill Livingstone, Edinburgh

Hadden D.R., Drury M.I., Kuhl C. & Molsted-Pedersen L. (1986). Three articles on pregnancy entitled Clinical controversy. *Diabetologia*, **29**, 1–16

19: Diabetes in Children

Childhood diabetes has a prevalence of 1 in 800 for the ages 0–15 in the UK. The disease is rare under the age of 5 and the incidence rises to a peak at 9–15 years of age.

Insulin-dependent diabetes in children is similar to the disease in adults though children are more likely to be HLA DR4 positive and to have insulin autoantibodies and very low insulin levels at the time of diagnosis. About 95% of children presenting with diabetes have IDD; however a few are NIDD and this is known as Maturity Onset Diabetes of the Young or MODY. Some children with MODY have a strong family history of the disease which appears to be inherited as an autosomal dominant; these children have 'Mason-type diabetes' named after one of the first families to be described (see p. 25). Children with NIDD must be identified since they can mistakenly be allocated to insulin treatment for the rest of their lives.

Neonatal diabetes is extremely rare. The babies are usually born to non-diabetic mothers; the child is often premature or immature at birth and fails to thrive. Despite adequate fluid replacement the child often loses weight and is dehydrated though not ketoacidotic. The diabetes responds to insulin treatment which can almost invariably be stopped after several months as the child starts secreting adequate amounts of endogenous insulin. The cause of this transient diabetes is unclear though it is generally believed to be due to slow maturation of the pancreatic insulin-secreting B-cells.

Clinical manifestations

Children usually present with the typical diabetic symptoms (see p. 8) of thirst, polyuria and weight loss. In addition they may present with secondary enuresis, abdominal pain, hyperventilation, perineal thrush, failure to thrive or failure to develop. As with IDD adults ketoacidosis is sometimes the mode of presentation. All these symptoms respond rapidly to control of the blood glucose.

Urinary problems

Persistent or recurrent enuresis is often a feature of poor diabetic control; it resolves when good diabetic control is achieved, sometimes with the help of a simple reward system, though more intensive management is required should the problem persist after the age of 6. Urinary tract infection is unusual in children and no more common in diabetic than in non-diabetic children. A urine infection confirmed by culture should be investigated further by an intravenous urography and a renal ultrasound. A micturating cystogram to exclude ureteric reflux should be performed in children under the age of 5 but in older children these investigations are only needed if the infection is recurrent or the other tests are abnormal.

Eating disorders

Eating disorders including anorexia and bulimia are thought to be more common in diabetic children, especially girls. Patients with such eating disorders can have considerable difficulty controlling their diabetes and it has been suggested, though not yet confirmed, that these diabetics are at high risk from diabetic complications. Young diabetics, particularly girls, are prone to an increase in skin-fold thickness associated with obesity. Obesity can become a problem as growth ceases at the end of puberty and weight continues to increase. Careful assessment of weight centiles should lead to early identification of this problem and dietary intervention.

Growth

Growth is a sensitive index of health. Most children with diabetes grow normally though some diabetics may lose about 2 inches in their final height, especially if they had poor glucose control while they were growing. Diabetics may also reach puberty 1 or 2 years later than is usual and pubertal delay causes loss of the pubertal growth spurt which exacerbates growth retardation. Normal height can still be attained due to more rapid growth than usual once puberty is initiated. It is important to identify delays in puberty and growth at an early stage and accurate height records are essential. Once a significant delay has been identified it should be investigated. Particular attention should be paid to the exclusion of hypothyroidism which is more common in young IDD patients than normal and almost impossible to detect clinically. A delay in puberty can be distressing for children and, even if no cause other than diabetes is found, the possibility of inducing puberty therapeutically should be considered.

Epilepsy

Children are prone to epileptic fits induced by factors such as fever or hypoglycaemia. Only if a child has more than one fit should they be investigated with an EEG. If the EEG is suggestive of an epileptic tendency it is our practice to start anti-epileptic treatment whilst carefully monitoring the blood drug levels since non-compliance is frequent. Treatment is continued for at least 2 years after fits have stopped.

Risk factors for complications

Blood pressure should be checked annually. Though hypertension is no more common in the early years of IDD than normal it may be an important risk factor leading to diabetic complications. The normal range for blood pressure in children differs markedly from that in adults and blood pressure centiles in children should be consulted. Smoking may be another important risk factor and children should be actively warned against it. Both drugs and alcohol can impair levels of consciousness and interfere with awareness of hypoglycaemia. Blood lipids should be checked if there is a family history of premature vascular disease or hyperlipidaemia.

Diabetic complications

Clinical complications are very rare in children and their appearance is closely related to the duration of diabetes.

Nephropathy

Up to 40% of young diabetics will develop diabetic nephropathy after 40 years of diabetes (see Chapter 13). Clinical proteinuria (>0.5 g/day) indicating diabetic nephropathy in IDD does not develop until diabetes has been present for at least 7 years and is uncommon before 15 years of diabetes. Identification of children at risk is not yet possible though there is a considerable research effort devoted to determining whether small amounts of protein in urine (microalbuminuria) presage clinical proteinuria. Proteinuria occurs transiently in both diabetic and non-diabetic children; such idiopathic transient proteinuria is benign, self-limiting and the commonest cause of proteinuria in children. Should proteinuria persist over 4 months then urine samples taken at bed-time and on rising should be tested to exclude orthostatic proteinuria and infection should be sought; haematuria or casts indicate a non-diabetic renal problem. The presence of haematuria or casts or an abnormal 24 hour urine protein (>140 mg/m^2/24 hours in children) should lead to an opinion from a nephrologist.

Retinopathy and cataracts

Diabetic retinopathy seldom develops in diabetic children within 5 years of diagnosis but most IDD patients will have some retinopathy after more than 20 years with the disease. Of these however only about 5% have visual impairment as a result of their diabetes — this never occurs before puberty.

Very rarely young diabetics develop bilateral cataracts shortly after the onset of the disease (see p. 140). These dense subcapsular or floccular cataracts form at the posterior pole in a few weeks leading to irreversible blindness. The cause of these cataracts is unknown; they do not appear to be related to poor diabetic control. They can be operated upon successfully.

Neuropathy

Diabetic neuropathy is seldom a clinical problem in children though changes in nerve function can be detected even before puberty. Congenital deformities of the feet such as pes cavus can be identified and advice should be given for chiropody and foot care.

Contraception

As girls attain an age when they may be sexually active they should receive advice on contraception. We recommend that diabetic girls use a low-oestrogen combined contraceptive pill; contraindications to its use are the same as in non-diabetics (see p. 203). As pregnancy in young girls is not uncommon, all girls who are menstruating should be counselled on the importance of diabetic control during the peri-conceptual period to reduce the rate of congenital malformations.

Management

Aims

The aim of management is that a child with diabetes should lead as normal a life as possible while achieving the best feasible diabetic control. This is a difficult target to achieve in practice due to modes of treatment and the need for glucose monitoring.

Acute management

The acutely-ill child requires urgent correction of dehydration and acidosis and the management is similar to that for an adult with ketoacidosis (see p. 96), though allowing for the difference in size. Fluid balance in a child must be meticulous and insulin, given intravenously if possible, can be given at an initial hourly rate of 0.1 U/kg body weight. If a newly-diagnosed child is not acidotic or severely ill we make every effort to manage them at home, not admitting them to hospital, and letting them return to school at the earliest opportunity.

Maintenance

Diabetes control can be maintained in young children on a single injection of insulin though twice daily injections are required as the child becomes older. Children under 9 years of age are, therefore, usually given a single morning injection of an intermediate-acting insulin, occasionally with the addition of a short-acting insulin. Children older than 9 years are, as a rule, given twice daily injections of insulin (both injections as either fast-acting or intermediate-acting or a mixture of the two). About 15% of children go through a 'honeymoon' period about 3 months from diagnosis when they have sufficient, though transient, recovery of B-cell function for them to stop insulin treatment for periods of a few months up to 2 years from diagnosis. It is our policy not to stop insulin during this period as it will inevitably need to be restarted and this return to insulin can be demoralizing. However, a flexible approach is best and in some cases insulin could be temporarily stopped. The insulin requirements rise progressively during childhood, usually remaining in the range 0.5–1.5 U/kg body weight. Puberty is associated with insulin resistance and the insulin requirements may rise sharply at that time.

It can be very upsetting for parents to give a child injections especially if the child dislikes them. One *must* be firm but never force the child. It may help the child to have a routine before giving the injection. Children can be encouraged to give their own insulin after they are 9 years old though some start at a younger age, but it is not necessary to insist as they all manage to do so eventually. Children who are reluctant to give their own injections gain considerably from holidays organized by the British Diabetic Association where they will meet other children who can cope.

There seem to be three major problems with insulin administration: (1) some children with poor diabetic control do not take all their insulin injections; (2) the injection technique may be incorrect; and (3) children often inject in a single site causing fat hypertrophy and, as a result, poor insulin absorption.

Oral hypoglycaemic agents are rarely used in children unless they have MODY. There is no particular preference for any particular agent in children but, if diabetic control can be maintained and growth and development is adequate, then there is no reason why a child on oral hypoglycaemic agents cannot remain on them. If control or growth does become inadequate then insulin should be started immediately.

Diet

The diet of a diabetic child should be tailored so that it resembles their previous eating habits and those of the family. In babies and infants normal feeds can be given while making appropriate adjustments to the insulin dose. Older children should avoid refined sugar and be encouraged to eat regularly. A carbohydrate exchange system can be introduced later. The amount of carbohydrate depends on the age, appetite and activity of the child; pre-pubertal children may require about 150 g carbohydrate per day as compared with adolescents who need up to 280 g daily. When the child stops growing and reduces exercise on leaving school the caloric intake should be reduced. Obese diabetic children must be encouraged to reduce their total calorie intake but not necessarily their carbohydrate portions; stringent weight reducing diets are not recommended. Before any exercise children must take extra carbohydrate — the amount depends on individual requirements and the type and length of exercise.

Hypoglycaemia

Hypoglycaemia is always a cause for concern among parents. It is important to reassure parents, and the child too, that however terrible the child may look during hypoglycaemia he will always wake up and he will neither die nor develop brain damage. The symptoms of hypoglycaemia in a child are the same as in an adult (see p. 109) though there are two other symptoms which may be (but not always) due to hypoglycaemia: naughtiness and bad temper. Some children think they are hypoglycaemic when they are only tired; others may say that they are hypoglycaemic when they want a sweet! If there is any doubt then it is important to measure the blood glucose. Finally children are prone to have fits when they become hypoglycaemic. If this happens more than once then they should have an EEG to exclude epilepsy as a cause of the fit.

The management of hypoglycaemic episodes is the same for children as for adults. Parents can give glucagon injections if the child loses consciousness though it is not routine to offer it to parents; it can be injected under the skin like insulin or into a muscle. Once the child recovers he should be given a snack to replenish the stores of hepatic glycogen and prevent recurrence of hypoglycaemia.

Assessment of control

Two categories of tests are used to assess diabetic control: (1) home testing of urine or blood glucose; and (2) clinic testing of glycated proteins. If the child is very young urine glucose can be tested by squeezing his nappy over a testing stick. Children over the age of 9 are encouraged to test themselves. Most children are very reluctant to do this during school; they can test at the week-end instead. Measurement of glycated proteins provide an index of diabetic control independent of the patient's assessment. Occasionally the child's estimate of control is different from the results of the glycated proteins: the former invariably suggests good control and the latter poor control. It is essential not to criticize the child or make them feel guilty about these discrepant results. There are three steps to be taken:

1   Confirm the discrepancy.

2   Exclude haemoglobin abnormality, for example persistent production of haemoglobin F which causes false elevation of haemoglobin A1.

3   Explain the apparent discrepancy to the parent and child and check their technique for testing. The discrepancy rarely persists!

Non-attenders

Some children fail to attend the clinic and in our experience of an inner city clinic, some 10% of the children (always adolescents) fail to re-attend. This group tend to be poorly-controlled diabetics often from difficult social circumstances. It is important to identify such individuals and to make every effort to establish contact with them as some of them can change their ways and be induced to re-attend regularly.

Development

Diabetic children are not more prone to psychiatric morbidity than normal individuals. Nevertheless there are many psychological and social pressures which might influence a child's development and attitude to diabetes. The attitude towards diabetes of the child, the siblings and parents, the school, friends and the doctors will all be important in determining how the child copes. The medical personnel looking after the child need to contact and educate these disparate groups; this means that the management of the child with diabetes is the work of a team.

Parents feel particularly responsible for children with diabetes. As the child grows up they have to allow them more responsibility; this transition can be very difficult but it must be done as adolescents resent interference by over-protective parents. Parents must also remember their responsibility for the other children who can feel left out if attention is focused solely on the diabetic child.

School

Diabetic children should not have to miss more school, apart from visits to the clinic, than any other child. They can undertake all the normal activities and their academic and sporting achievements should not be diminished. The diabetes specialist nurse from the clinic should visit the school as the child may be the only diabetic they have, and they will naturally be nervous about the condition and their responsibilities. The nurse will talk to the class teacher and the school head, secretary, nurse and cook, dealing with the following points:

1 The need for mid-morning and afternoon snacks.

2 The teacher's responsibility to ensure that the child has lunch (which should preferably be selected from normal school food).

3 The teacher should know how to recognize and treat hypoglycaemia.

4 Sport should be encouraged with the usual precautions, including extra carbohydrate beforehand.

5 Swimming is allowed but each diabetic child must be supervised by a teacher.

6 The child is encouraged to go on school trips — the British Diabetic Association provides a 'school pack' for teachers supervising these trips. The Association also organizes camps for diabetic children during the holidays which are a wonderful opportunity for children with diabetes to meet each other.

Manipulation

Diabetes provides an excellent opportunity for manipulation (see also p. 86). It is normal for all of us to try to manipulate situations to our personal advantage. It is important to appreciate what is happening. Diabetes should not be an excuse to live differently from everyone else. This point is as important for the child who tries to manipulate his parents or teachers as it is for the over-protective parents who try to stop their child living normally. Exploitation of illness follows a pattern in children as well as in adults and includes psychosomatic symptoms, malingering, self-poisoning, Munchausen syndrome and non-compliance. The last of these leads to non-attendance, falsification of tests and failure to take insulin. At worst these diabetics may have their lives disrupted by multiple episodes of diabetic ketoacidosis, or more rarely, severe hypoglycaemia; they are usually adolescent girls on large doses of insulin and known to a number of hospitals.

Despite the range of problems outlined above the majority of diabetic children cope remarkably well and lead an essentially normal life.

Further reading

Baum J.D. & Kinmonth A-L. (1986). *Care of the Child with Diabetes*. Churchill Livingstone, Edinburgh.

20: Spontaneous and Reactive Hypoglycaemia

Diabetologists are occasionally asked to see non-diabetic patients with hypoglycaemia, usually to exclude an insulinoma.

Hypoglycaemia is generally defined as a blood glucose of 2.2 mmol/l or less. The normal fasting blood glucose after a 24-hour fast in women is lower (mean 3.5 mmol/l) than in men (4.0 mmol/l), though these levels fall further with prolonged starvation.

In diabetic patients, by far the commonest cause is excessive insulin or sulphonylurea therapy sometimes precipitated by inadequate food intake (p. 111) but there are many other possible, if rare, causes for its occurrence in non-diabetics. There are listed in Table 20.1.

The most important distinction is between fasting and reactive hypoglycaemia, as the causes, pathophysiology and investigation of the two groups are completely different. The distinction should be obvious from the history.

Fasting ('spontaneous') hypoglycaemia

As the name implies, the condition is characterized by hypoglycaemia occurring in the fasting state; this is nearly always apparent in the history where relief of the symptoms after food is characteristic. The symptoms themselves may be very varied, ranging from altered consciousness and bizarre behaviour to cardiovascular collapse. Attacks are occasionally provoked by exercise.

Investigation

Laboratory blood samples should always be taken during symptoms and before administration of glucose; blood sticks are not accurate in this range, even with a meter.

Hypoglycaemia must be proved (<2.2 mmol/l) before the differential diagnosis is considered. This is best done by three overnight fasts (15 hours in duration); samples for glucose and insulin are taken at the end, or earlier if the fast has to be terminated; insulin is only estimated if glucose is low.

Table 20.1 Possible causes of 'spontaneous' hypoglycaemia

Pancreatic
  Insulinomas
  Nesidioblastosis
Endocrine deficiency
  Primary hypoadrenalism
  Hypopituitarism
Drugs
  Alcohol
  Insulin   ⎱ Especially in medical personnel
  Sulphonylureas ⎰   and relatives/friends of diabetics
  Salicylates
  Paracetamol
Inborn errors of metabolism
  e.g. glycogen storage diseases
  Leucine, galactose, fructose sensitivity
Hepatic failure
Infections
  Malaria
Other tumours
  Fibrosarcoma, especially retroperitoneal
  Hepatoma

The next consideration is whether, at the time of hypoglycaemia, plasma insulin is suppressed, as it should be, or inappropriately raised. The 'appropriate' range for plasma insulin and blood glucose is shown in Fig. 20.1; subjects with insulinoma have inappropriate insulin levels for the glucose. These tests detect about 90% of insulinomas, the classical cause of fasting hypoglycaemia in the absence of other systemic disease in the adult. Insulinomas (islet-cell tumours) were first recognized in the 1920s when they were shown to contain large amounts of insulin; soon afterwards surgical removal was shown to cure the condition.

C peptide estimation distinguishes factitious hypoglycaemia in which it is suppressed from insulinoma in which it is increased in parallel with insulin. Plasma proinsulin may also be elevated in patients with an insulinoma. Anatomical localization methods include angiography, CT scanning, which often does not detect these small tumours, and portal venous sampling for insulin.

Other causes are discovered by assessment of clinical symptoms, signs and appropriate investigations.

Treatment

Treatment of insulinomas should be surgical when possible, though symptomatic treatment may include diazoxide (5 mg/kg body weight in

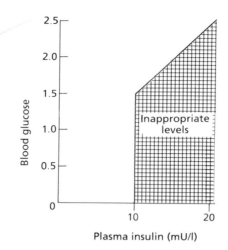

Fig. 20.1 The appropriate range of plasma insulin for given levels of fasting hypoglycaemia.

two or three doses initially) with or without a thiazide diuretic (e.g. bendrofluazide up to 10 mg/day). Malignant lesions may be treated with streptozotocin and 5-fluorouracil or by hepatic embolization; a somatostatin analogue has also been used for symptomatic control.

Treatment of other causes is that of the underlying condition.

'Reactive' hypoglycaemia

This occurs 2–4 hours after a meal. The appropriate investigation is a prolonged 4–5-hour oral glucose tolerance test, which shows a fall below 2.2 mmol/l — a fall to 2.5 mmol/l is normal at 90–150 minutes after a 75 g OGTT.

The commonest cause of reactive hypoglycaemia is after gastric surgery, where rapid food transit times cause excessive release of insulin. It may also occur just before the diagnosis of diabetes.

The diagnosis of 'reactive' hypoglycaemia is frequently made in the USA on the basis of doubtful and inadequate blood glucose data. It is rarely, if ever, the cause of vague post-prandial symptoms.

Further reading

Marks V. & Rose F.C. (1981). *Hypoglycaemia*, 2nd edn. Blackwell Scientific Publications, Oxford.

Section 5
Diabetic Care

21: The Organization of Diabetic Care

Introduction

Care of diabetic patients requires enthusiasm and organization and, above all, a team of experts working closely together, hospital specialists linking with general practitioners. Details will differ between districts and there can be no claim to a universal perfect model. The geography and distances of travel will alter the preferred plan of service as do the standard, interest and facilities of the hospital specialist and general practitoners. The BDA has issued recommended levels of staffing and minimum advised standards.

For obvious reasons the discussion is biased towards arrangements for an inner-city teaching hospital district with a major district hospital function! The principles however apply more widely.

The diabetes centre

An area in, or close to, hospital should be set aside for diabetic care — whether or not it is named as such, this should become the Diabetes Centre. An essential part of diabetic care is the immediate availability of advice for those in difficulties at any time of day, and preferably at nights and weekends as well. The facility for patients to be seen quickly is vital and, during normal hours, there needs to be a 'help-line' telephone answered by a sensible, trained and sympathetic person with access to appropriate advice; the number should be widely publicized. Outside conventional hours calls should be transferred to an appropriate person, a designated trained nurse or doctor member of the team.

Within the centre there should be facilities for education of both patients and staff with regular meetings for both audit purposes and to maintain interest. Rapid provision of advice to other firms and departments within the hospital must also be available.

The concept of the Diabetes Centre has developed from these requirements and its purposes may be defined as follows:

1 Availability of advice at all times, not limited to those of conventional diabetic clinics.

2 The centre of organization of district diabetes services and coordination with general practitioner shared care or Mini-Clinic schemes.

3   The home of a register, preferably including all diabetic patients in the
district and not just hospital patients. This allows the facilities to be offered
to all.
4   A centre of education resources and programmes for patients and staff,
including community-based nursing staff.

The team

A wide range of trained specialists is needed to give comprehensive care to
diabetic patients: they include hospital physicians and general practitioners,
specialist health visitors and nurses, dietitians and chiropodists. A
dedicated ophthalmologist, obstetrician and orthopaedic and vascular
surgeons familiar with the special problems of diabetes should be part of the
team. If a district nephrologist is not available there should be close liaison
with the regional centre(s).

The diabetic specialist nurse and health visitor

The most important single innovation in diabetic care during the past three
decades has been the increasing involvement of health visitors and sisters
with special expertise in the care of diabetics. An enthusiastic health visitor
or sister transforms the standard of diabetic care, achieving liaison between
hospital, general practitioner and patients at home and offering a wide
range of clinical and educational expertise. Most normal-size districts will
need two or more full-time specialists.

The training of nurses for diabetes care is of central importance and is
undertaken both in the clinics themselves and at specially designed day-
release courses (in Britain Course ENB 928 organized by the Clinical Board
of Nursing Studies).

Diabetic services

However the district services are organized, wide-ranging services are
needed which include:
1   Routine care with management and control of diabetes.
2   Screening and detection of complications.
3   Treatment of complications.
4   Care of those who are acutely or chronically ill.

These aspects of diabetic care are undertaken at the Diabetes Centre, in
diabetic out-patient clinics and in a small number of in-patient beds. They
may also involve shared-care schemes and mini-clinics as well as
community care facilities. Exact arrangements will vary in different districts.

These functions determine the siting of the Diabetes Centre which should be organized as an independent unit preferably within, or at least very close to, the local acute hospital. The centre should include consulting rooms, educational areas, offices for staff, dietetic and chiropody facilities and a clinical laboratory.

Special diabetic services

EYE CLINICS

Facilities for regular testing of visual acuity and examination of fundi through dilated pupils (using tropicamide 1% for mydriasis) in a darkened room need to be available. Ideally diabetic clinics should run in parallel with an ophthalmology clinic with an interested specialist who has access to laser photocoagulation treatment (Chapter 14). If this is not possible foolproof and rapid referral arrangements must be made.

ANTENATAL CLINICS

Clinics in which the diabetic physician(s) see patients jointly with a single obstetrician who has developed a special interest in this field have been responsible for major advances (Chapter 18). Where this is not possible close liaison is essential; neonatal paediatricians also need to be involved.

DIABETIC FOOT CLINICS

These need to take care of education and prevention with routine chiropody, as well as treatment of those with ulceration and sepsis (Chapter 17). Facilities for neurological examination and Doppler examination of the circulation are needed. Where the population is very large, clinics may be divided into those with neuropathic and those with ischaemic problems (p. 172). Above all, immediate access for those developing an acute problem is absolutely essential and can often prevent the development of overwhelming disease. A shoe fitter or orthotist should attend regularly and needs some simple facilities for making adjustments to shoes and insoles (grinder, oven).

DIABETIC RENAL CLINICS

Facilities are now needed for the detection of nephropathy so that appropriate investigations and treatment are undertaken (Chapter 13). As renal function deteriorates collaboration with a renal physician becomes important and ideally larger centres should run joint clinics for these patients. An introduction to the renal unit and its staff is offered before end-stage renal failure develops so that patients are prepared well in advance. In districts without this expertise mechanisms must be devised to allow rapid referral before severe symptomatic renal failure is reached.

CHILDREN AND TEENAGERS

Requirements for the care of diabetic children are amongst the most difficult to organize and vary widely between isolated paediatricians with no diabetic input and the reverse (Chapter 19). The team needs most of the same skills as an adult clinic (dietician, specialist nurse) but social workers are valuable additional members. Considerable social and family support is needed and liaison with schools is essential.

The needs of teenagers are even more delicate and their disinclination to attend hospital clinics probably understandable. Organization of their care in unconventional ways is best undertaken by those skilled in caring for this group of young people.

Education

An integral aspect of diabetes care is to inform all patients of the nature of the disorder and its treatment and to place the potential threat of complications in their true perspective. Educational facilities are offered by the whole diabetic team both to individuals and groups.

The aims of an education programme are:

1   To explain the nature of the disease and its complications.
2   To explain the treatment, starting with the simplest ground rules and eventually providing comprehensive instructions on both treatment and monitoring.
3   To explain dietary requirements.
4   To provide printed literature. Our 'starter' packs contain:
       a booklet about diabetes,
       dietary instructions,
       home monitoring booklet with full instructions,
       essential telephone numbers,
       leaflets on the British Diabetic Association.

Instructions to new patients are always given initially on an individual basis. Most centres also organize courses for groups, ranging from a single half-day to comprehensive weekly series. These should be different for IDD and NIDD patients and should provide scope for discussion and questions as well as direct instruction.

Education of patients has become very sophisticated in the field of diabetes; it has reduced admissions and to some extent complication rates, notably amputations. It is a concept which could be applied much more extensively to other areas of medicine.

Records

Special records are needed for proper care of diabetic patients both in hospital and in general practice — however this is organized, they must be immediately available when required. In hospital there are huge advantages in maintaining a separate set of records for diabetics and this system is used in many major departments. Many general practices also keep special records supplementary to the basic 'Lloyd-George' card. Such records must be designed for serial recording of factual data, weight, blood glucose, blood pressure, urine tests, haemoglobin A1, visual acuity, complications (results of eye examination in particular) and treatment (Fig. 21.1). There must always be space for the normal recording of the medical consultation itself and for treatment recommendations.

There should be a system to alert the staff to the presence of particular problems, for example, sight-threatening retinopathy, and to the date when the next examination is required (for example blood pressure or eye examination). Many also incorporate an education check-list which records when patients have attended sessions and ensures that essential advice has been given (e.g. driving). Some examples of these records are shown in Table 21.2.

Computers are invaluable for maintenance of good records on diabetes, though no single system is clearly superior. Maintenance of a complete register of diabetic patients is a simple and essential operation; records of varying complexity can also be held on the computer and the presentation can be structured so as to present the necessary information described above. There is a danger of printing excessive amounts of detail which only confuse and obscure important information.

Links with general practice

'Shared care'

Care of diabetic patients is best conducted in a co-ordinated way linking the hospital clinic and the general practitioner's surgery. It requires enthusiasm at both ends and in general practice it is ideal if one member of the practice is chiefly responsible for the organization. Patients are best seen in specially organized clinics so that the necessary facilities can be brought together — dietitian, chiropodist, specialist nurse, visual acuity test, urine and blood glucose tests. Special records (Figs 21.1 & 21.2) are needed in general

CAMBERWELL SHARED CARE SCHEME

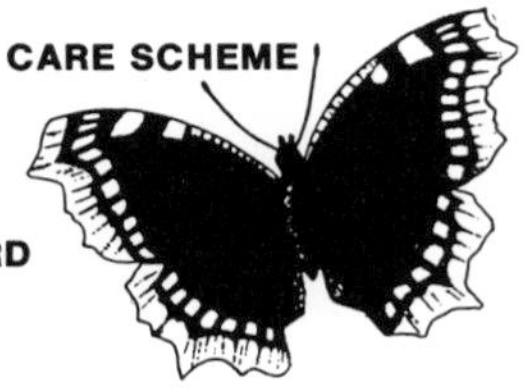

DIABETIC RECORD CARD

Name: ....

Address: ....

....

....

Tel No: ....

GP Name: ....

Address: ....

....

Tel No: ....

Diabetic Clinic
King's College Hospital, London SE5 9RS
(Dr P.J. Watkins and Dr P.L. Drury)

Hospital number: ....

Special notes:

PLEASE BRING THIS BOOK AND ALL YOUR TABLETS WITH YOU AT
EVERY VISIT TO SURGERY OR CLINIC

Produced jointly with the Camberwell Primary Care
Development Project

Fig. 21.1 Part of the record card valuable in the shared care scheme.

practice as they are in hospital and the concept of the shared care book maintains the link.

In most centres the majority of new patients are generally diagnosed, examined, registered and taught about their diabetes in the hospital clinic. Once appropriate treatment is established, patients attend their general practitioners (where defaulting rates are less) and perhaps return for major review and assessment in the hospital clinic perhaps on an annual basis. Patients suitable for shared care will vary with the expertise and interest of the general practitioner, the distance travelled and the wishes of the patient. Hard and fast rules are neither appropriate nor desirable. Children, pregnant women and those with major complications are normally seen at hospital clinics.

Because problems may arise acutely, the hospital clinic must have

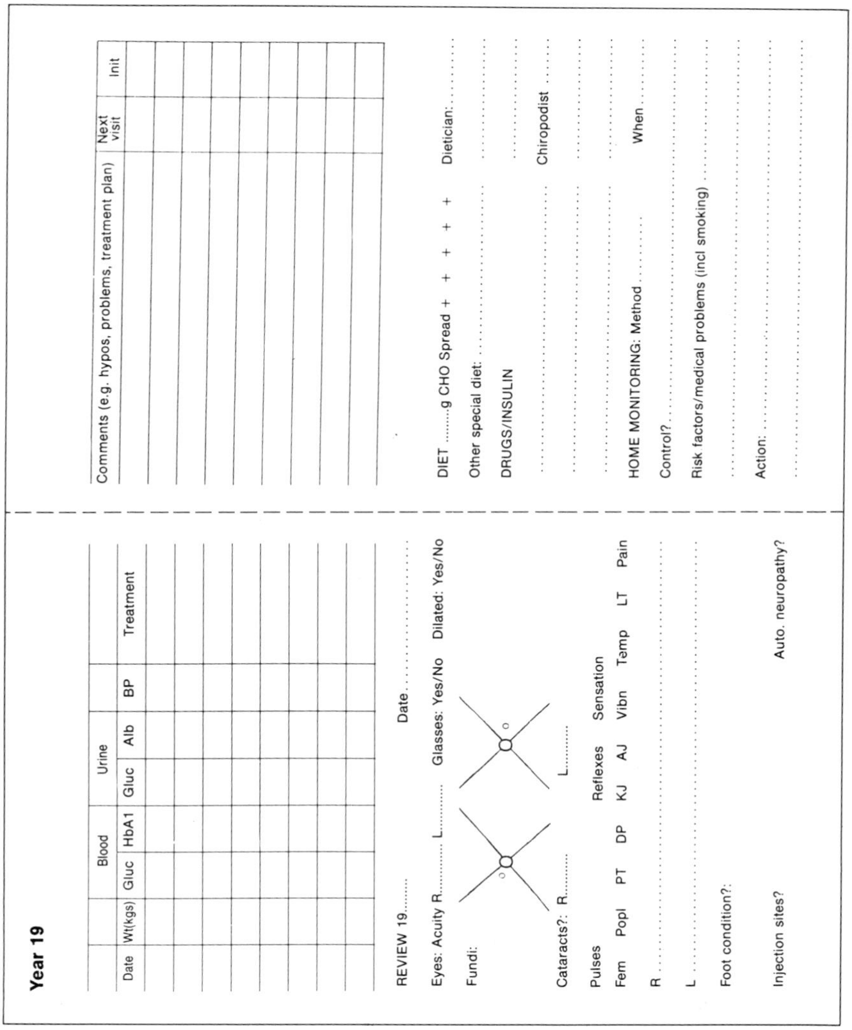

Year 19

| Date | Wt(kgs) | Blood | | Urine | | BP | Treatment |
		Gluc	HbA1	Gluc	Alb		

Comments (e.g. hypos, problems, treatment plan)	Next visit	Init

REVIEW 19........   Date ....

Eyes: Acuity R........... L.......   Glasses: Yes/No   Dilated: Yes/No

Fundi:

Cataracts?: R.............   L.............

Pulses   Reflexes   Sensation
Fem Popl PT DP   KJ AJ   Vibn Temp LT   Pain

R ....

L ....

Foot condition?: ....   Auto. neuropathy?

Injection sites?

DIET ....g CHO Spread + + + + +   Dietician: ....

Other special diet: ....

DRUGS/INSULIN ....   Chiropodist ....

....

HOME MONITORING: Method ....   When ....

Control? ....

Risk factors/medical problems (incl smoking) ....

....

Action: ....

Fig. 21.2 Part of the record card used in the shared care scheme.

arrangements for seeing patients immediately if the general practitioner seeks urgent advice; this is an essential part of shared care. Good schemes provide the best standards of diabetic care, the most agreeable conditions for patients and the lowest defaulting rates. There is however a constant need to nurture the scheme in order to maintain interest and standards, and regular meetings are undertaken, every few months, for audit, exchange of information, presentation of cases and provision of new information. The greatest concern of most GPs is the adequacy of their retinal examinations.

'Mini-Clinics'

In some centres local GPs and the consultant(s) have arranged satellite 'mini-clinics' where intermittent visits to interested practices allow him/her to see difficult cases, advise on general policy and pass on new information and techniques. While outstandingly successful in a few centres, it requires great commitment from all involved.

Audit

However services are arranged, the aim must be to deliver care to the whole diabetic population. While sometimes it is the patient presenting with advanced retinopathy or renal failure who is to blame for avoiding or ignoring advice, it is still too often the fault of individual doctors or health personnel, or of the organization of care. Regular audit, including an investigation of apparent failures such as amputation or blindness, is an essential requirement for maintaining and improving standards of diabetic care.

Further reading

See Appendix reading list on p. 236.

22: Social and Legal Consequences of Diabetes

Introduction

Most of the problems of diabetic patients in society result from the ever-present possibility of hypoglycaemia in insulin-treated diabetics. Lack of public understanding is a real problem, together with the erroneous notion that most diabetics may be crippled by complications of their disease. This often results in unwarranted bias against them in both work and leisure activities. These problems can often be solved by good sense on the part of the diabetic and those he lives and works with. The British Diabetic Association is always worth consulting in case of difficulty (see Appendix).

Employment and leisure activities

The guiding principle in making the difficult assessments for employment or leisure activities is whether the risk of confusion during hypoglycaemia affects the individual only, or whether it also places the safety of others at risk.

Individual organizations generally have their own guidelines regarding the suitability of diabetic patients for particular activities. If candidates are rejected unreasonably they may appeal. Diabetic patients are not normally accepted by the armed forces, the police, the merchant navy or the fire brigade; they may not serve as pilots. There are some restrictions on driving (see below). Shift work, especially night-shift work, should be avoided if possible by those on insulin, but sensible diabetic patients can make appropriate adjustments and may successfully cope with such work. Some leisure activities are obviously risky, including mountaineering and scuba diving (the latter not usually allowed) where the hazards can be very great.

Diabetic patients who are treated by diet alone or with oral hypoglycaemic agents and who are otherwise fit should be permitted to undertake any occupation or hobby. Their risk of hypoglycaemia is very small.

Driving

Ordinary driving licences can be held by diabetic patients whether on insulin or not provided that they are otherwise physically fit and not suffering from blackouts. The present law requires that all diabetic patients, regardless of their type of treatment, should inform the Department of Transport (DVLC, Swansea). When they apply for a driving licence for the first time, diabetes must be declared on the application form; it is helpful to indicate whether or not insulin is being used. Driving licences are issued for 3 years and then renewed (at no extra fee) subject to a satisfactory medical report.

Insulin-treated diabetics may not hold public service and should not hold heavy goods vehicle licences because of the serious potential consequences of hypoglycaemia, no matter how small the risk may be to the individual. Healthy diabetics not needing insulin are normally allowed to hold these licences, though some transport employers do not permit the use of sulphonylureas.

Avoidable accidents still occur in diabetics who become hypoglycaemic while driving. It is essential that they should follow guidelines to make driving safe and to maintain a good reputation for the diabetic driver. Thus, they should never drive if they are late for a meal when the danger of hypoglycaemia is particularly great; the latter half of the morning may be a dangerous time for this. Many patients will now measure their blood glucose before driving, especially if there is some doubt at the time. Failure to use home blood glucose monitoring will become increasingly difficult to defend. Diabetics should always keep a supply of sugar within immediate reach in their cars. If they do experience warning symptoms of hypoglycaemia they should stop, switch off the ignition and leave the car since they are otherwise open to a charge of driving under the influence of drugs (insulin). They should take sugar and then wait 10–15 minutes, or at least until the symptoms have completely disappeared. Those unfortunate diabetic patients who are prone to disabling hypoglycaemic attacks without warning must not drive.

As with all applicants for driving licences, satisfactory vision is essential; those with marked impairment may not drive.

Insurance and pensions

Driving insurance with a normal premium should be issued subject to a satisfactory medical report; of course, diabetes must be declared. Life assurance premiums are often raised by amounts which depend on the result of a medical examination. Sickness and holiday insurance premiums are also likely to be higher than normal. The British Diabetic Association offers helpful advice.

Patients who are registered blind are eligible for supplementary pensions. There is sometimes difficulty in obtaining jobs with firms which have superannuation schemes for their employees. In a large firm there should be little trouble but the extra hazards for a diabetic, especially in terms of life cover, may deter a small business employer.

Travel

Diabetes control is easily upset by the rigours of travelling. Regular monitoring needs to be undertaken and appropriate adjustments made to the insulin dose. Dieting easily goes astray and changes of activity, which may be more or less than normal, can lead to hypoglycaemia or hyperglycaemia respectively. Ample equipment and insulin should be taken and always kept with hand baggage, never in an aircraft hold. Insulin will keep for some months at room temperature in temperate climates, but should be kept in a refrigerator in tropical climates; it should never be deep-frozen. Inoculations should be given as for non-diabetics.

Measures described on p. 86 should be adopted if vomiting begins, and insulin maintained throughout. The usual anti-emetics can be used, including those used for motion sickness; apart from causing some drowsiness they do not interfere with diabetes control.

Time changes on long-distance air travel inevitably cause some disturbance of diabetic control for a few days. When travelling from east to west, the day is lengthened and supplementary amounts of soluble insulin (perhaps 4–8 units) may be needed to tide the patient over until his next regular insulin injection is due. Conversely, travelling from west to east, the shorter day may necessitate either additional carbohydrate or a small reduction of the insulin dose. Blood testing should be performed more frequently.

Dental treatment

Dental treatment should not be affected by diabetes, nor is there any good evidence that dental or gum disease is exacerbated by diabetes. Treatment under local anaesthetic is carried out as normal, but when general anaesthesia is needed, a brief hospital admission is wise for insulin-treated diabetics, and measures are taken as described on p. 107.

Legal aspects

Diabetes and legal questions arise chiefly in relation to driving (see p. 227), behaviour and actions during hypoglycaemia, and in relation to the medico-legal question whether trauma or accidents may cause diabetes.

Trauma

There is nothing to support the notion that the trauma causes diabetes, and abdominal injuries sufficiently severe to cause permanent pancreatic damage would scarcely be compatible with life. Difficulties do arise nevertheless when diabetes is discovered after an accident. A doctor may then be asked by lawyers not whether diabetes has been caused by the accident, but whether he can be certain that it has not. Although one may feel confident that it is much more likely than not that no relationship exists, it can still be difficult to assert that there is none. In most cases there is no definite proof that the patient did not have diabetes before the accident. There is, however, always the possibility that trauma may have precipitated clinical diabetes rather than caused it. Signs of retinopathy or other long-term complications may prove that the diabetes was present long before the injury. When the onset of clinical diabetes follows closely — in a matter of days rather than weeks — after the injury, speculation with regard to a relationship is even more difficult.

In established diabetes, trauma frequently causes a deterioration of control, which is however always temporary.

Hypoglycaemia

Hypoglycaemia is one of several causes of 'automatism' which is defined as 'the existence in any person of behaviour of which he is unaware and over which he has no conscious control'. During this state criminal acts may be performed especially shoplifting, driving offences and breaches of the peace.

A person can be guilty of crime only if he has engaged in a certain conduct (*acta reus*) with a certain state of mind (*mens rea*), the latter indicating guilty intent and implying that the individual committed the crime of his own volition. An automaton-like state relieves the offender of '*mens rea*' (the guilty intent) and can be advanced as a defence to criminal charges. In practice this means that if the presence of hypoglycaemia at the time of the act can be established, some offenders are successfully acquitted.

Lawyers are however cautious in their use of this defence because of the readiness with which it might be abused. Furthermore, if it can be shown that the hypoglycaemic state was the result either of carelessness or even deliberately induced, it can cease to be a valid defence.

The law regarding automatism is however extremely confused. A defence of automatism strictly means that a state of insanity, albeit temporary, must be pleaded: the outcome of such a verdict might be committal to an institution for mentally ill offenders which would scarcely be sensible in a case of hypoglycaemia. Further discussion of these legal points will be found in the article below.

Further reading

Frier B.M. & Maller G. (1988). Diabetes and hypoglycaemia: medico-legal aspects of criminal responsibility. *Diabetic Medicine*, **5**, 521–526

Appendix and Useful Information

Equipment for injection of insulin

Insulin 'pen' devices

These deliver metered doses of insulin from an insulin cartridge. They are portable and greatly simplify the procedure of measuring and administering insulin. The insulin dose is either pre-set on a dial, or measured by delivering the appropriate number of clicks on the plunger. These devices are very convenient for those who are blind or partially-sighted. It is likely that 'pens' will gain in popularity and gradually displace the conventional insulin syringe.

Soluble insulins are already available in cartridge form, and insulin mixtures of short- and medium-acting insulins will shortly be available.

Some insulin 'pens' are: Novo Pen, Insuject (UK licence pending), Accupen.

Syringes

Plastic syringes with needle attached are the most convenient. Needles are very fine (27 g) and usually 1/2 inch. Patients using less than 50 units at a single injection (i.e. the majority) should use a 0.5 ml syringe (total capacity 50 units) since the marking is much clearer than on the 1 ml (100 unit capacity) syringe. These syringes can be used several times. The needles should be covered with the plastic cap, and units should preferably be kept in a refrigerator; they should never be stored in spirit.

Pre-set syringes

Traditional glass syringes are still available with a screw-locking device which can be set at any required dose. This technique is still valuable for those who experience difficulty with measuring their insulin dose.

Click-count syringe

The plunger of this glass syringe has a ratchet mechanism which enables the dose to be measured by clicks. It is not easy to use.

Table A.1 Insulin infusion pumps

	Graseby MS36	Nordisk Infuser
Address	Graseby Medical Colonial Way Watford Herts	Nordisk UK Nordisk House Garland Court Garland Road East Grinstead W. Sussex
Size (mm)	120 x 58 x 25	100 x 60 x 20
Weight (g)	170	180
Appearance	Smart	White metal, clinical
Reservoir insulin	2 ml syringe (Graseby)	Prefilled cartridge Velosulin 570 U
Basal range (U/24 hours)	1–99 In 1 unit steps	7.5–100 In steps
Bolus control	Push-button tactile + audible feedback, 1 unit	Push-botton 1 unit
Power	Disposable 5.4 V battery	Disposable 5.4 V battery
Battery life	10 weeks	28 days
Alarms	Full	No blockage/empty reservoir

Insulin pumps

Several suitable infusion pumps are available. They infuse insulin at a basal rate and have facilities for delivering a pre-prandial boost either manually or electronically. The pump is usually worn in a pouch attached to a belt around the waist or a shoulder harness. There are two pumps which are at present generally used in the UK; details are shown in Table A.1.

Monitoring equipment

Blood glucose

Blood is obtained by pricking a finger, usually to one side of the nail, or (a little more painfully) on the pulp itself, or (with difficulty but painlessly) the ear lobe. The equipment required is: (1) finger pricker; (2) blood glucose test strip; and (3) some patients like to use a blood glucose meter but it is not essential.

1 *Finger pricker.* A spring loaded pricker is best since its use results in a sufficient quantity of blood and it is virtually painless. It uses a purpose-made disposable needle (e.g. Monolet). Examples of good finger prickers include:

Autolet (Owen Mumford Ltd)
Monojector Lancet Device (Sherwood Medical, Crawley, Sussex)
Autoclix (Hypoguard, Woodbridge, Suffolk)
Glucolet (Ames Division, Slough).

2 *Blood glucose test strips.* The test strips are read by eye or by meter. The following strips are available:

BM–Test Glycemie 1–44
Ames Visidex II
Ames Glucostix
Hypoguard GA Test Strips.

It is very important to remember that blood glucose readings at the top of the scale of each of the strips represent minimum values and actual blood glucose levels could be much higher. All these strips can be obtained on prescription.

3 *Blood glucose meters.* Several meters are available at prices of £40–80 (1989 prices). The most recent development which is likely to prove very successful is a pen-sized device, the ExacTech Blood Glucose Meter (Baxter Healthcare Ltd, Unicare Medical Services Ltd, Cambridge Road, Harlow, Essex): the sensitive area of the strip containing the enzyme remains outside the instrument, no washing is required, and the reading is obtained in 30 seconds. At present the strips are expensive and are now obtainable on prescription. Other meters use some of the strips described above and several of them have a built-in memory of 10–40 previous results. The Glucochek meter (Medistron Ltd, Horsham West Sussex) retains the previous 400 blood glucose values; blood glucose profiles can be printed using the Glucocheck printer. Other systems (for example, Hypocount MX, Hypoguard, Woodbridge, Suffolk) have smaller memory systems recording the previous ten blood glucose results.

4 *Capillary blood samples.* If patients cannot cope with self-measurement of blood glucose but can manage to take capillary blood they can take their samples to hospital in simple plastic tubes coated with heparin and fluoride (Sarstedt tubes) and have their home blood glucose profiles measured at the diabetic clinic.

Urine testing equipment

Urine tests for glucose are usually performed using paper strips although some patients still prefer the older Clinitest tablet method.

1 *Glucose test strips.* There are several including diastix (glucose 1/10–2%), Diabur 500 (1/10–5%). Glucose readings by diastix are to some extent reduced by the presence of ketones.

2 *Urine tests for the blind.* The Hypotest meter reads the diastix strip and gives an audible signal indicating the amount of glycosuria.

3 *Clinitest tablets.* These record positive results to all reducing agents, which in most cases indicates the presence of glucose. The test is to some extent inhibited by vitamin C (ascorbic acid). When very heavy glycosuria is present, the colour change tends to go through orange (2%) and back to green (1%) which can be misleading.

4 *Ketone strips.* Patients are not normally asked to test urine for ketones, although when illness supervenes the presence of ketonuria adds a sense of urgency to treatment. Only a modest increase of blood ketones is needed for the urine to become strongly positive. Ketostix is usually used. Ketostix can also be used for plasma tests: a ++ or +++ reaction in plasma establishes the presence of ketoacidosis.

5 *Albumin.* Patients are not normally requested to test for albumin. Albustix is used in most clinics and starts to record positive tests at approximately 150 mg/l.

Sensory testing: vibration sensation

The Biothesiometer (Biomedical Instruments, Newbury, Ohio, USA) is a satisfactory instrument only if it is carefully used by a single observer. The test can be performed on the tip of the big toe, the dorsum of the foot or at the malleolus; the same site should always be used. Three readings should be taken. Readings are in 'volts'. A reading of more than 10 V at the big toe is usually abnormal, and if it is over 35 V there is a risk of ulceration. There is some deterioration with age.

The calibrated tuning fork may be more satisfactory and it is much cheaper.

Aids for impotence

These function by applying a negative pressure to the penis which results in an inflow of blood and thus erection. They are worn like a condom, and there are various methods of generating a vacuum. They are relatively expensive and not suitable for all cases.

The Correctaid is obtainable from Genesis Medical Ltd, Freepost 24, London W1E 5HP. Most of the purchase sum is refundable if the device proves unsatisfactory.

Educational material

Every new patient should be supplied with a packet containing material which describes diabetes together with its problems and treatment. IDD and NIDD patients of course need different information. It should contain:

An account of diabetes management (specific for IDD/NIDD)

Problems of hypoglycaemia (for IDD)

Diet (specific for the individual)

Monitoring techniques (blood glucose or urine testing)

Foot care.

Many publications are available; a wide variety can be obtained from the British Diabetic Association (BDA).

Publications from the BDA

A catalogue is available, but the following are useful titles:

Insulin-Dependent Diabetes, by J.L. Day (1986).

Non-Insulin-Dependent Diabetes, by J.L. Day (1986).

Countdown (a guide to carbohydrate and calorie values of manufactured foods and drinks).

Many cookery books.

A wide range of leaflets are also available on many aspects of diabetes.

Other publications

Day J.L. (1986). *The Diabetes Handbook: Insulin-Dependent Diabetes.* Thorsons Publishing Group, Wellingborough in collaboration with the BDA, London

Day J.L. (1986). *The Diabetes Handbook: Non-Insulin-Dependent Diabetes.* Thorsons Publishing Group, Wellingborough in collaboration with the BDA, London

Diabetes: a Practical Guide for Patients on Insulin, by R. Tattersall. Churchill Livingstone, Edinburgh (1986).

Knowing about Diabetes: for Insulin Dependent Diabetics, by P.H. Wise. W. Foulsham & Co. Ltd, London (1983).

Knowing about Diabetes: for Non-Insulin Dependent Diabetes, by P.H. Wise. W. Foulsham & Co. Ltd, London (1983).

Coping with Life on Insulin, by J.M. Steel & M. Dunn. Chambers, Edinburgh (1987).

Diabetes: a Beyond Basics Guide, by R. Hillson. MacDonald Optima, MacDonald & Co. Ltd (1987).

The Diabetes Reference Book, by P.H, Sonksen, C. Fox & S. Judd. Harper & Row, London (1985).

The Diabetic Child, by J.W. Farquhar. Churchill Livingstone, Edinburgh (1981).

Diabetes in your Teens, by J.W. Farquhar. Churchill Livingstone, Edinburgh (1982).

Other items available for diabetics

FOR THE VISUALLY HANDICAPPED

Cook books on cassette — from the BDA
Leaflets on diet in braille — from the BDA.

VIDEOS

A wide range of instructive videos can be purchased or hired from the BDA.

IDENTITY ITEMS

Medic-Alert bracelets from Medic-Alert Foundation, 11–13 Clifton Terrace, London N4 3JP.

INSURANCE

The BDA advises on all forms of insurance. In particular, patients can contact H. Stephenson & Co. Ltd at C1 Tower, St George's Square, New Malden, Surrey KT3 4HH (tel. 01 336 2000).

Tables for ideal body weight

	Men			Women	
Height (cm)	Ideal weight (kg)	120% (kg)	Height (cm)	Ideal weight (kg)	120% (kg)
155	56	67	144	46	55
156	56	67	145	46	55
157	57	68	146	47	56
158	58	69	147	47	57
159	58	70	148	48	58
160	59	71	149	48	58
161	59	71	150	49	59
162	60	72	151	49	59
163	61	73	152	50	60
164	61	73	153	50	60
165	62	74	154	51	61
166	62	75	155	51	61
167	63	76	156	52	62
168	64	77	157	52	63
169	65	78	158	53	64
170	66	79	159	54	65
171	66	79	160	54	65
172	67	80	161	55	66
173	68	81	162	55	66
174	68	82	163	56	67
175	69	83	164	57	68
176	70	84	165	58	69
177	71	85	166	58	70
178	71	86	167	59	71
179	72	87	168	60	72
180	73	88	169	61	73
181	74	89	170	61	73
182	75	90	171	62	74
183	76	91	172	63	75
184	76	92	173	63	76
185	77	93	174	64	77
186	78	94	175	65	78
187	79	95	176	65	78
188	80	96	177	66	79
189	81	97	178	67	80
190	82	98	179	68	82

Diabetic associations

British Diabetic Association

10 Queen Anne Street
London W1M 0BD
Telephone 01 323 1531

The American Diabetes Association

1660 Duke Street
Alexandria
Virginia 22314
USA

Juvenile Diabetes Foundation

60 Madison Avenue
New York, NY 10010
USA

National Diabetes Information Clearing
House

Box NDIC
Bethesda, MD 20205
USA

The Canadian Diabetes Association
(National Office)

78 Bond Street
Toronto
Ontario M5B 2J8
Canada

The Diabetic Association of
New South Wales

250 Pitt Street
Sydney
New South Wales 2000
Australia

General Reading List

Alberti K.G.M.M. & Krall L.P. (1984–1989). *Diabetes Annual*, Vols 1–5. Elsevier, Amsterdam

(*A series of brief reviews of topics of recent interest and advances within diabetes.*)

Besser G.M., Bodansky H.J. & Cudworth A.G. (1988). *Clinical Diabetes: An Illustrated Text.* J.B. Lippincott, Philadelphia

(*A fully-illustrated handbook of diabetes with explanatory text.*)

Bliss M. (1983). *The Discovery of Insulin.* Paul Harris Publishing, Edinburgh

(*A masterful account of the events surrounding the discovery.*)

Bloom A. & Ireland J. (1980). *A Colour Atlas of Diabetes.* Wolfe Medical Publishers, London

(*A cheaper atlas of well-chosen illustrations.*)

Brownlee M. (ed) (1981). *Diabetes Mellitus*, Vols I–V John Wiley, Chichester

(*Multivolume textbook covering both biochemical and clinical aspects of diabetes.*)

Draznin B., Melmed S. & LeRoith D. (eds.) (1989). Complications of diabetes mellitus. *Molecular and Cellular Biology of Diabetes Mellitus*, Vol. III. Alan R. Liss Inc., New York

The Diabetes Handbook: Insulin-Dependent Diabetes, by J.L. Day. Thorsons Publishing Group, Wellingborough in collaboration with the BDA, London (1986).

The Diabetes Handbook: Non-Insulin-Dependent Diabetes, by J.L. Day. Thorsons Publishing Group, Wellingborough in collaboration with the BDA, London (1986).

(*Two handbooks for patients, but with much practical information of use to clinicians.*)

Ellenberg M. & Rifkin H. (eds) (1983). *Diabetes Mellitus: theory and practice*, 3rd edn. Medical Examination Publishing, New Hyde Park, New York

(*Well-known American textbook.*)

Gale E.A.M. & Tattersall R.B. (1989). *Diabetes — the Art of Clinical Management*. Churchill Livingstone, Edinburgh, in press

(*Comprehensive multi-author handbook of practical management of diabetes.*)

Keen H. & Jarrett J. (eds) (1982). *Complications of Diabetes.* Arnold, London

(*Outstanding source book on the microvascular complications.*)

Leslie R.D.G. (1989). Diabetes. *British Medical Bulletin,* **45**. Churchill Livingstone, Edinburgh

(*Recent series of concise articles on many aspects of diabetes.*)

Marble A., Krall L.B. & Bradley R.F. (eds) (1985). *Joslin's Diabetes Mellitus,* 12th edn. Lea & Febiger, Philadelphia

(*One of the definitive American textbooks.*)

Nattrass M. (ed) (1983, 1986). *Recent Advances in Diabetes,* Vols 1–2. Churchill Livingstone, Edinburgh

(*Series of well-referenced reviews on selected aspects of diabetes.*)

Nattrass M. & Hale P.J. (eds) (1988). *Non-Insulin Dependent Diabetes. Bailliere's Clinical Endocrinology and Metabolism,* Vol. 2.

(*Single volume with reviews of all aspects of NIDD.*)

Watkins P.J. (ed) (1986). Long-term complications of diabetes. *Clinics in Endocrinology and Metabolism* **16**, 715–1003.

(*Single issue with well-referenced reviews of the microvascular complications.*)

West K.M. (1978). *Epidemiology of Diabetes and its Vascular Lesions.* Elsevier, New York

(*Despite its age, a classic review of diabetes in a world setting.*)

World Health Organization (1980). *Expert Committee on Diabetes Mellitus. Second Report.* Technical Report Series No. 646. WHO, Geneva

World Health Organization (1985). *Diabetes Mellitus.* Technical Report Series No. 727. WHO, Geneva

(*Two WHO reports including diagnostic criteria. Committee style, but full of facts and figures.*)

Index

Page references in *italic* indicate figures and/or tables